The Carnivore Diet

A Complete Beginner's Guide To Get Lean, Get Ripped, and Lose Fat with 30 Easy Keto Recipes

Grant Matthews

Table of Contents

Introduction 1

Chapter 1: A History Of Carnivorous Food........... 3

Chapter 2: What Is The Carnivore Diet? 9

Chapter 3: How Does This Diet Work?.................18

Chapter 4: What to Eat And What To Avoid 28

Chapter 5: Pros And Cons Of The Carnivore Diet.37

Chapter 6: Differences Between The Carnivore Diet, Keto, And The Paleo Diet 41

Chapter 7: Who Is The Carnivore Diet For? 53

Chapter 8: Carnivore Diet Tips for Success.......... 61

Chapter 9: 30 Easy Carnivore/Keto Recipes 74

Breakfast 74

1. Easy-peasy egg and cheese sandwiches:..................74

2. Healthy Toad in a Hole: 75

3. Jalapeno and egg bacon cups 76

4. Healthy Breakfast Hash 77

5. Low Carb Breakfast Pizza.......................................78

6. The Dreamy Breakfast Tower 79

7. Bacon and Egg Roll-Ups 80

8. Eggs in Purgatory..82

9. Eggs in Heaven..83

10. Steak and eggs...84

Dinner...85

1. Shrimp scampi with zucchini zoodles.....................85

2. Roasted chicken...86

3. Pan-roasted duck breast with butternut squash.....87

4. Grilled chicken hearts and livers............................89

5. Burger bombs...89

6. Flat iron steak with caramelized onions.................90

7. Oven-roasted Salmon with Pesto...........................91

8. Pan-roasted scallops with asparagus......................92

9. Roasted chicken thighs with tomato and jalapeno salsa...93

10. Perfect filet mignon with roasted mushroom sauce
....95

Dessert...96

1. Blueberry Tarts..96

2. Individual Pumpkin Tarts......................................98

3. Chunky chocolate chip cookies..............................99

4. Individual chocolate tarts.....................................100

5. Pecan Cookies...102

6. Chocolate Mug Cake.................................... 103

7. Peanut Butter Pie 104

8. Chocolate-chip Cheesecake 105

9. Pound cake with lemon frosting........................... 107

10. Key Lime Pie... 109

Final Thoughts **111**

Introduction

Congratulations on downloading your copy of *The Carnivore Diet* and thank you! I am pleased to help you navigate your way through to your best self with The Carnivore Diet. Also known as the zero-crab diet, this meat-lover's utopia is a tool for weight loss. Some people have even reported it as a means to address autoimmune conditions. We will explore defining your goals and taking steps to achieve success using meal plans and providing you with the knowledge to make the right choices.

This e-book will guide you through the information you need to reach your personal goals using The Carnivore Diet. We will walk you through every aspect of beginning this diet, from the history of the food that makes up the carnivorous diet, to the pros and cons of the diet, and finally, we will end with some recipes and some final thoughts on this diet.

We will also spend some time talking about diet culture and what it means to actually be on a diet. We will explore how to be successful on this or any diet and help you to really identify why you want to go on this journey and make sure that you are in the right frame of mind before you start this journey.

Each recipe will include instructions for preparation, ingredients, and cooking times. Hopefully, all of this information will help you make the best personal choices for your taste and lifestyle. We have ten breakfast recipes, ten dinner recipes, and ten dessert recipes. We think they are all pretty fantastic recipes and think you will too. These are easy recipes, so even if you can barely boil water, we are confident that you can make these recipes and enjoy a delicious meal in no time at all.

Many books are dedicated to The Carnivore Diet and so thank you very much for making this selection as your go-to for a guide on The Carnivore Diet. The objective is always to include as much fruitful information as you need to make your goals a reality.

Go forth and devour your goals!

Chapter 1: A History Of Carnivorous Food

Ever since the first human slopped out of the proverbial ooze, meat has been an integral part of our diet. Humans over millennia evolved into quite the effective hunter – with our sharp bicuspids, our large brains, and opposable thumbs. We are smart, we can effectively tear things apart with our hands, and our teeth are sharp enough (or used to be anyway) to pierce flesh.

Our ancestors had diets made almost entirely out of meat. I personally have this scene from Ice Age playing out in my head where a human with entirely too much hair by modern standards decides to try to take out a mastodon so that he and the rest of the tribe can eat for the rest of the winter. But lest you think that this entire book is going to be based on an animated children's movie, let me tell you that there are several solid examples of indigenous peoples surviving on entirely on game and living long and healthy lives. I am going to take you through several examples: the Inuit, the Chukotka, and the Maasai people.

The Inuit people live in the Arctic. As you can imagine, not a whole lot grows up there. It is literally a frozen wasteland much of the time, and where there is soil, it usually does not grow things that are fit for human consumption. So what is left? Game meat and what you can catch from the sea. The Inuit people have survived for centuries on seal, walrus, moose, caribou, and reindeer. They, of course, would also occasionally eat whale meat, salmon, whitefish, ducks, geese, and sometimes ptarmigan.

Starting to get the picture? Not a lot of vegetation or fruit in sight. Yet these are some of the healthiest people on the planet! This phenomenon has often been called a "paradox". Modern science keeps trying to tell us that a diet heavy in meats and fats is going to kill us because it will raise our blood pressure to unhealthy levels and clog our arteries with a lack of fiber. Yet the Inuit people defy every finding from those studies. Of course, the Inuit people probably don't smoke, spend 17 hours a day in front of technology, and drink themselves silly on the weekends. In other words, what I'm trying to tell you here is that while their dietary choices obviously make for a big part of their health, so do other decisions in their every day lives.

One of those decisions is whether to eat processed foods. Macaroni and cheese that came in a box was simply not an option for our ancestors and neither was it an option for the indigenous Inuit people. In fact, pretty much any processed food you can think of was never a part of the human diet right up until the 1950s, which is when the world's health started to take a deep decline. You didn't find our hunter-gatherer ancestors sitting by the fire stuffing their faces with prepackaged cakes, cookies, and cereals. They had diets rich in protein and fat. There really is something to that.

But the Inuit are not the only indigenous people who have survived for centuries on a high fat, high protein diet. The Chukotka natives of Russia also have survived for centuries on caribou, seal, salmon, and other varieties of fish. They also would quite often use seal oil or hot caribou fat to cook their food or drizzle on top of fish much like we would dress a salad with olive oil. Several studies have been done regarding the Chukotka peoples' health, and again, their health is exemplary. Nary an example of poor heart health or cancer due to a diet high in protein and fat and low in carbohydrates.

Speaking of fat, let's take a moment to discuss this most magical of substances. When you eat a diet that is high in protein, you must accompany it with enough fat. There are a plethora of examples of people dying because they ate protein that was too lean and nothing else. Your body needs fat in order to survive. Plain and simple. Not to mention that eating fat will help you feel fuller for longer, which will help you feel nice and satiated even when "on a diet." We will talk a little bit more about what it means to be on a diet later in the book. For now, we would like to move on to the Maasai people of Africa.

I was first introduced to the Maasai people when I was watching an episode of Anthony Bourdain's (may he rest in peace) "Part's Unknown." In the episode, Tony was taking a tour through Tanzania and was lucky enough to get to meet with this tribe of excellent people. As he was wont to do, because it was what he loved and because it was what he was good at, he talked with these tribesmen about their diets.

So, a little bit on who the Maasai are: a native tribe in Tanzania who consider themselves to be stewards of the world's cattle population and who regard themselves as the mortal enemy of the lion. I mean, I don't know about you, but while I fear lions like any sane person, I don't necessarily think enough of myself to consider the lion my mortal enemy. Then again, I don't rely on lions leaving my herds alone so that I can earn a livelihood. Anyway, long story short – they are a fierce, fierce people. They have fought lions and come out victors – often with a lion pelt to prove their prowess as warriors. So when they give advice on diet and exercise, I feel like it's worth a listen. Maybe I can turn into the kind of warrior that will make lions run. Even if I don't, losing some weight and being able to run really fast will be a pretty cool side-effect.

And their diets consist of meat, milk (fermented – kind of like yogurt), and blood. Yeah, blood. I'm not recommending that you go out and fill up your water bottle with the blood of freshly slaughtered animals. But what I am suggesting is that this is yet another indigenous tribe that survives almost entirely on a high protein and high fat with no serious health consequences. In fact, the Maasai people have near super-human cardiovascular capacities and can keep pace with Olympic athletes.

At the end of the day, remember that our ancestors did not have access to a Whole Foods every 30 miles. Food production was limited to either what they or their village could catch and cook. Or sometimes gather. But it took a lot more effort to gather and cook vegetables and fruit than it did to take down one big animal, preserve its flesh, and then cook it as needed.

Our ancestors did not rely on protein powders or big protein bars to get their nutrients. And in fact, their systems could probably not have tolerated those food products due to all the chemicals that are now in them. It is no coincidence that cancer rates have been on the rise since preservatives and other chemical additives have been introduced to the supply chain. Allow me to go on a small rant about the current state of our food chain.

Bread is not supposed to last for a week on the shelf. Fruit is not supposed to be covered in wax – it's not a candle. Food that we eat is not supposed to have ingredients in it that we cannot pronounce. Even before I adopted this particular diet, I had a rule about packaged foods: if it had more than five ingredients or any ingredient at all that I could not pronounce, it did not make its way into my cart. And then when I started doing more research on diets like the carnivore diet and the paleo diet, I started to see how many things are added to our food that one, do not need to be there, and two, that can also cause us great harm.

No, our ancestors did not live to be 100 years old. But I would argue, quite convincingly, I think, that their lifespans were not shortened because of their diets. Their lifespans were short because they were constantly exposed to the elements, they did not have proper medical care (i.e., vaccines, routine doctor visits, antibiotics, etc.), and because they had not established themselves as the predator at the top of the food chain yet. If mastodons and saber toothed tigers were still running around Manhattan, I think we would struggle to keep our average lifespan up around the mid-eighties.

So our history of food is eating what the earth gives us. The earth gives us whole, nutritionally dense food that gives us all the nutrition we need. We do not need to seek help from supplements, powders, or chemicals. We have everything we need right in front of us.

So what does this history mean for me?

In short, it means that you, as a human being, are uniquely suited for a diet high in fat and protein with little to no carbohydrates. The thing is, while scientists and nutritionists have continuously harped on the idea that we need a diet that is diverse in order to cover all of our nutritional bases. But it looks like all of the research may not have been necessary.

Chapter 2: What Is The Carnivore Diet?

The Carnivore Diet is exactly what it sounds like, really: a diet based entirely around eating things that were formerly swimming, walking, or flying. This diet is based on the idea that a diet high in protein and fat is going to be far healthier for you than any other kind of diet. This is because our ancestors survived on diets very similar to this – they ate diets comprised almost entirely of protein and fat, with very little vegetation and fruit.

The reason for this is that our ancestors tended to live in places where either a lot of vegetation didn't grow or where it would be extremely inefficient to go out and try to get enough green stuff to keep them alive. So they focused on meat, which gave them the most caloric bang for their buck. And that still holds true today!

See, the reason why meat is a better vehicle for all of those micronutrients is because of something called "bioavailability." So, whenever we eat plants, we are not just directly absorbing the nutrients that they have. More often than not, we have to convert different molecules in the plants into other...different molecules. I'm not a scientist, but what I'm trying to say here is that it takes a lot of effort for us to turn plants into nutrients that we can use.

Well, what's wrong with plants?

Honestly, we are not anti-plant around here. We don't have our offices stripped bare of any plant life and we do eat the occasional salad when we feel the urge. But 99% of the time we eat only meat and fat. Not only does it taste good, but it provides us with the micronutrients that we need to be fully functional humans. We are going to go through a few micronutrients that humans need and explain why plants are not necessarily the best source for those nutrients.

Vitamin A

Vitamin A is a nutrient that plays a big part in our memory function, our ability to learn, and is also very important for our eyes! I don't know about you, but I grew up with my grandparents chasing me around with carrots, insisting that if I didn't eat them, I would go blind. And yet, here I am, many (many)years later and still not blind because I didn't eat the silly carrots.

Because here's a secret – carrots don't actually have any vitamin A at all! What they actually have are molecules called caretonoids, which then get turned into vitamin A when we chew and digest plant foods, like carrots. But it is plentiful in meat, and much more easily absorbed by our systems when it is taken from meat as well.

Vitamin D

I remember being pregnant with my son and panicking. I was panicking for a lot of reasons, but chief among them was making sure that my growing boy was getting enough Vitamin D. I live in a place where it is not easy for me to get a lot of sunshine, and I burn like a lobster anyway – so vitamin D is difficult for me to produce just by going outside. So I was forced to consider other sources.

Vitamin D is absolutely essential for our brains. We need it from the beginning in order to fully form our brains, we need it to help support our brain's memory capacity, and we need it to help keep our brain safe as it ages. Obviously, this is a really important micronutrient! And the way my doctor talked, I was either going to have to eat roughly a truckload of broccoli or swallow some horse pills to get enough Vitamin D for myself and my new addition.

Neither of those options sounded particularly appetizing to me, so I did some research. What I found, again, was that Vitamin D is much more bioavailable from meat sources. So I ate some more protein and fat and my boy is healthy, smart, and cute. I don't think Vitamin D helped him get cuter, but it sure is a bonus that he's so cute. Especially when he destroys my house.

Vitamin K2

Vitamin K...what? I hear you asking, you in the back. Yeah, I didn't know what this particular micronutrient was either until I went ahead and adopted the carnivore diet. Turns out this is a super important micronutrient that helps our brain cells to form their membranes and just generally keeps our brain safe and healthy.

A safe and healthy brain, especially as I age, is very important to me. So when I found out that vitamin K2 is absent from any and all plant foods. But it is abundant in foods sourced from animals. So it's really a no-brainer. (See what I did there.)

Vitamin B12

This is another vital micronutrient that is not readily available through plant sources. Vitamin B is used to made DNA, RNA, red blood cells, and myelin, which insulates the pathways between our brain neurons. Again, this is a clearly important micronutrient that we need in our diets. In diets that are entirely plant-based, people can have very serious vitamin B deficiencies, which in extreme cases can lead to death.

But this vitamin is present in animal foods in abundance. It is most concentrated in clams and beef liver, both of which are included in the carnivore diet plan. This is good news for your energy levels and your red blood cells!

Iodine

Again, when I was pregnant with my son, I was very concerned about his well-being. That meant I needed to be sure that I was getting the appropriate amounts of micronutrients in my diet. One of those essential micronutrients is iodine. I have a thyroid problem and so iodine is even more important to me.

Lack of iodine can lead to poor brain development and can even stunt growth. Obviously, I wanted to make sure that my developing son would have enough iodine to support his stay in my body and then be ready when he came earthside. So I made sure I ate enough meat and also had enough table salt in my diet. Table salt is treated with iodine, which helps ensure that people get enough iodine in their diets.

Zinc

Remember those tablets your mom used to make you swallow at the first sign of a cold? She said that they were zinc tablets and would make sure that you were well enough to go to school the next day. Boy did I hate those things. At the first sign of illness, my mom would just pile those things in my hands and watch me until I took every last one of them. Of course, I was then able to go to school, instead of staying home and watching "The Price is Right."

Bitter childhood memories aside, zinc is actually really good for you. It helps your immune system, it boosts your vitamin B6 production and also helps you make serotonin, which is the chemical in your brain that helps keep you happy. I don't know about you, but I like being happy.

Unfortunately for vegetarians and vegans, plants are notoriously low in zinc. But meat, particularly beef, is an exemplary source of zinc. Not to mention that it will be a whole lot easier for you to absorb the zinc that comes from meat versus the little bit that comes from plant life.

Omega-3 Fatty Acids

Omega-3 fatty acids are the main support systems for our immune systems and for our brain functions. Our brain requires DHA, which helps to make those sheaths around our neurons and helps to keep brain membranes healthy. DHA is also used when our brain forms new pathways, which is why it is so important for young children to get DHA in their diets. For example, when you look at prenatal vitamins, they are often advertised as being fortified with enough DHA and EPA for healthy fetal development.

Those who eat diets comprised entirely of plants or diets that consist mainly of plants with supplements of eggs and dairy, they are missing out almost entirely on DHA and EPA. Food sources that are particularly rich in these fatty acids are oily fish like salmon and foods such as liver and other animal organs. So it's one of the many benefits of this diet that you will expose yourself to this much-needed micronutrient that helps support a healthy brain and immune system.

As you can clearly see, there are so many vital micronutrients that are easily available in a carnivorous diet! It can be difficult to get many of these micronutrients from a plant based diet, particularly because it can be very difficult for humans to break down the different molecules in the plant-based foods and then actually absorb them.

Okay, but what exactly do I eat?

We have another section of the book where we will go through a list of foods and even give you some of the nutrient breakdowns. But just to give you an idea, this is not a diet for vegans or vegetarians. One hundred percent of your food intake will be from animals, including birds and fish. No tofu will be found in any of our recipes, and neither will grains, legumes, fruits, or vegetables. You will find a little bit of dairy (sometimes, but if you are lactose intolerant, please ignore those foods and skip the dairy. Nobody needs those uncomfortable feelings in their tummy.), and some odd herbs and spices, but that's about it.

Yes, there are plant foods out there that are sources of protein, but none of them are complete sources of protein. So we will not have any recipes here that feature peanuts or beans of any kind. Not only are these incomplete sources of protein, but they have also been shown to be gut irritants. Which is fun for no one, by the way. This diet is trying to make you feel better, not irritate your largest organ system.

But as I also said before, this diet will have some herbs and spices. This is for several reasons – one, it makes food taste better. As you can probably guess, eating meat and only meat will get a bit repetitive for a while, but herbs and spices will help mix things up and keep your palate excited.

Look, plants are not evil. They are not something that is going to kill you. But in the past few years, there has been such a push to eliminate meat from the human diet that we are dangerously close to having more and more people abandon meat entirely and thus eliminate essential micronutrients from their diets. We understand that plants can be tasty and sometimes can provide a nice balancing point in a diet. We are not suggesting that you eliminate plant foods from your diet forever. That just is nonsensical.

Do you see where I am going with this? It never makes sense to completely eliminate one food group forever and ever, bar none. I mean, if we are being honest, I am going to have some cake when it's my son's birthday. Is it healthy? No. Is it good for me? No. Will it fix all the problems in my life? No. But it does taste really good and it will make me happy for those few minutes that I get to sit down and enjoy it.

So just like we are telling you that it isn't realistic to eliminate plants and plant-based foods from your diet forever, we hope you see how equally ridiculous it sounds to completely eliminate animal products from your diet for the rest of your life. After all, what would the Fourth of July be without a big, fat, juicy steak on the grill? What would breakfast be without some bacon or a few sausage links? Boring and a whole lot less tasty, that's what. So remember, we are focusing here on not eliminating entire food groups for the rest of your life.

The purpose of this diet is to jump start weight loss and to help you start to make better choices for your diet. Remember, this is a diet that is based on choices that our ancestors would have made regarding food. They would not have had access to processed foods – and you can see that they had fewer incidents of cancer and other metabolic diseases. Rates of metabolic disease, including cancer, have been on the rise since the globalization of industrial food products.

Our ancestors ate whole, unprocessed foods that came from the earth. And that is the main theory behind this diet and the lessons that you are meant to carry forth as you move on in your life. Make choices to eat whole, nutritionally dense foods that are as close to the earth as you can get. This diet is not necessarily meant for you to follow for the rest of your life unless you so choose.

This diet is supposed to help jump-start weight loss. Follow this diet for 30-90 days and see how you feel. Make sure you take measurements and keep a journal – this will help you track your progress and will help you remember the potential roadblocks you may come across and how you overcame them.

Chapter 3: How Does This Diet Work?

The good news is, this is a pretty simple diet, but there are a few rules that you are going to need to follow in order to be successful. And these aren't just food rules either – these are rules that are going to help you become an overall healthier and happier human. Earlier we talked about the fact that we will help you discover your reasons and your goals with this diet and we are keeping that promise. This section of the book isn't just going to talk about the rules of the carnivore diet. We are going to do an in-depth overview of diets, diet culture, and what it means to try to change your life. We will give you the very easy-to-follow rules at the end of this chapter.

Diet Culture

Okay, so what does that even mean? Is it just one of those phrases that self-help gurus and life coaches like to toss around like so much fluff? No, it is a real thing. Diet culture is the backbone of the health supplements industry as well as the bodybuilding industry. People go on diets for so many reasons: whether it be to look a certain way to go on stage and compete, to fix something in their life that they know is missing, or to satisfy the person in the mirror. It is so important to understand that while there are many different motivations behind starting a diet, so many of them are unhealthy.

Diet culture is found in those Instagram captions you see where there is a girl with an impossibly tiny waist, round behind, and thighs that somehow manage to carry all that behind but still have a thigh gap. Oh, and her eyebrows, skin, and nails are absolutely perfect too. And it doesn't stop at women – men are absolutely victimized as well. Men are absolutely deluged with photos of sweaty, tanned men with perfect abs and the shoulders of Adonis. Men and women are constantly told that they are not enough, that they don't look quite right, that if they just had a six pack, as well as a six-figure income and perfect teeth, life would be just fine.

None of these marketing messages is aimed at actually making your life better. That Instagram model doesn't know your name, or care about your birthday, or know that you have a million other things that you need to worry about in your life besides the fact that your sixth ab just won't appear. But that's why we are here. We understand that when you make a major lifestyle change like choosing to follow the Carnivore Diet, you aren't just trying to change your appearance, you're trying to change your life. And we are here to help.

Well, a six pack is great. And a benefit to a great diet (cough, cough, like the carnivore diet!) But, when you start any sort of diet, you need to understand the motivations that you have. So maybe take five minutes right now, grab a piece of paper or one of your kids' discarded notebooks, and journal about why you want to start this diet. Talk about why you want to change your life and why you feel like you are finally ready to make this commitment to yourself. Ready? Go.

...Are you back? Good. What did you find out about yourself? Something good, I hope. So now that you have identified why you are doing this and why now is the right time for you, let's think about how you will keep yourself accountable during this journey. Because motivation is great for posters and for Mondays, but it is something that will dry up eventually. You need to get into the habit of treating yourself well. You need to get in the habit of eating well. You need to get into the habit of exercising.

Habits are what will take you far, no matter what goal it is you have. Habits are particularly important with this diet and lifestyle because, after a while, it can get rather repetitive. So if you are just in the habit of eating a lot of protein and a good amount of fat, it won't seem so repetitive and it won't seem like a chore. When things like good eating choices and exercise are just a natural part of the day, it doesn't become something you *have* to do, it is just something that comes as naturally to you as breathing.

Unique Benefits to the Carnivore Diet

As you can imagine, the whole reason why we wrote this book is that there are benefits to this diet. We didn't decide to devote hours upon hours of our time and energy just to write a book about a diet that doesn't benefit anyone. We figured that would be a waste of time for you and for us. So in this particular section of the book, we are going to talk about the different benefits to this diet and let you know what you have to look forward to as you become ever more carnivorous.

1. Weight loss: obviously, most people go on a diet so that they can lose weight. The nice thing about this particular

diet is that the weight seems to come off so easily. Like we have mentioned, when you are on this diet, you really aren't counting calories. You are just eating when you're hungry and eating until you're full. Whereas most of us can eat a whole bunch of snack foods in one sitting, it's very hard to eat a bunch of steaks without feeling ill. Also, protein and fats are excellent for satiety purposes. So you're not going to be feeling hungry all the time anyway.

2. You will enjoy better cardiovascular health. ...I know, I know. I can hear you wondering out loud how a diet filled with meat and meat products could possibly be good for your health. Well, believe it or not, science cannot tell you that your saturated fat levels will increase your risk of a heart attack. Instead, several studies show that increased levels of saturated fats can, in fact, increase your cardiovascular health.

3. Lowered levels of inflammation. One of the main culprits of inflammation in modern diets is legumes, grains, and nuts. Nuts and legumes can put a lot of stress on your intestinal system, as do grains. We also are becoming increasingly familiar with gluten as another cause of joint inflammation. Gluten can also cause some very serious side effects in those who are allergic, including anaphylactic shock.

4. Men have seen increased levels of testosterone. Ladies, this may not mean a whole lot to you, but it does mean that you will have to keep an eye on your testosterone levels with your doctor.

5. Improved digestion. Like we mentioned above, so many things that modern humans eat irritates our digestive systems. Grains and legumes are some of the main culprits of digestion upset. Fruit can also be a culprit – I think quite a few people know the effects of apple juice on a child's digestive system when they are constipated. Too much fruit can cause digestive distress.

These are just a few of the benefits of this particular diet.

So how do I change my life?

So that's the beautiful thing about realizing that you aren't going to follow diet culture and instead live and eat well to improve yourself just for *you*. When you do that, you are able to change your life in any way you choose. Honestly, nothing is impossible once you realize that you can do whatever it is you set your power behind.

To change your life, all you need to do is decide. Decide that this is no longer going to be a "one day" situation – that today is day one of your new life. Once you decide, really decide, that you are going to get healthy and lose weight, nothing can stop you. But I have a feeling that you're going to need more than just a few words on how to decide to change your life and maybe need a few concrete steps. What follows are five steps to weight-loss success that will help you shed pounds, get ripped, and change your life forever:

1. Decide that today is the day that your life changes. Get up, make your bed, and clear out your refrigerator and your pantry. You don't have time in your life for Rice Krispy treats anymore. Out of sight, out of mind.

2. Get some exercise equipment or join a gym. There are certain gyms out there that are only $10 a month to join. Just skip the pizza and bagels that they offer to their members for some inexplicable reason.

   a. I guess this is technically another step, but I consider it part of the whole "go join a gym" tip – you have to actually go to the gym or work out on your own. Go lift some weights, run a little on the treadmill, or swim. I don't really care how you do it, but you need to get in at least 30 minutes of exercise every day. You don't need to be like The Rock and get up at 4 AM and feel like you're going to drown in your own sweat every day, but at least 5 days out of 7, you need to break a sweat. On those other two days, do something a little less intense, but it is still important to get in physical exercise on those days.

3. Make your food list and go shopping. This book has a detailed food list detailing what you can and cannot eat on this diet. Copy down what you can eat and go buy it.

4. Buy some Tupperware that actually has lids that match – this will come in handy when you need to pack your breakfasts and lunches for going to work. I don't know about you, but I can't really grill up a steak at my desk.

5. Meal prep! This is going to be THE KEY as far as your success in this diet and in life. Every Sunday, or whatever day you have the most time, you need to gather your supplies and cook up big batches of food to store in your fridge for the week. So, make one or two of the recipes that we have listed here, let them cool, pop them in your containers, and then take them with you as the week goes on. This will help keep you on track and take the stress out of figuring out what to eat every day.

The Carnivore Diet- How to Follow It

Like I said before, this diet is really super simple. You want to focus on eating meats that are high in protein and high in fat. As long as it was once walking, swimming, or flying – you can eat it. Vegetarians can argue all they want that beans and nuts are good sources of protein, but that simply will not fly on this diet. As we have mentioned before, humans are not always so good at converting these plant foods into useful energy and absorbing the nutrients held inside these plants. So, we turn to animal protein.

Animal protein is a rich source of vitamins, minerals, and of course, amino acids. Amino acids are beautiful little building blocks for protein. Protein makes up so much of our body – we literally cannot function without it. And when we lack amino acids, our body can't make protein. Get my drift here? It's all a big circle and it begins and ends with protein!

So, if it once flew, swam, or walked, it's on the menu. Beef steaks, bacon, game birds, game meat, etc. This is not the section of the book where we go over the list of foods that are allowed versus foods that are not allowed, but hopefully, you are starting to get the idea. No plant foods or fruits are allowed on this diet. You can eat whatever you want, so long as it was once alive.

You might be wondering about supplementation and calorie counting. Well, on this particular diet, we do not really focus on counting calories. The idea here is that you are building up sustainable habits for the rest of your life, right? So we want to take this opportunity to encourage you to start listening to your body and only eating when you are well and truly hungry. This means that when it is time to eat, remove all the distractions. Don't text on your phone or mindlessly watch television – really pay attention to what you are eating. Eat slowly and mindfully. Actually, chew your food. You will be amazed at how little you actually eat when you really pay attention to your food and the act of eating.

So the long and the short of it is that on this diet, you really aren't going to be counting calories. You're just going to eat when you're hungry and stop when you're full. Simple as that. Now, let's talk about supplements. If you choose to supplement your diet because you feel like you are not getting everything you need, we understand. But not all supplements come in pills, remember! When you are on this all protein, high fat diet, it is really important to remember that you cannot just eat one type of meat – you have to mix it up.

So, what do you need to make sure you're eating and maybe supplementing? Make sure you are getting enough magnesium. This little micronutrient helps you with everything from making sure you are sleeping enough to making and keeping your bones strong. Magnesium is found in animal products, but your body may need more. You can pick up magnesium supplements in any health food store.

Regarding the foods you need to make sure you are incorporating into your diet, you need to make sure you are eating sufficient amounts of eggs, liver, seafood, spices/seasonings, and bone/collagen broth. Okay, so eggs are important for their fat content and the other minerals that they contain. Liver will help you make sure you are getting some Vitamin D, A, copper, choline, folate, and iron. It's kind of like the superfood of the animal world. Plus, it's absolutely delicious, so enjoy.

Seafood has tons of Vitamin D, selenium, copper, iodine, manganese, and iron – lots of awesome micronutrients that you need. Plus, it has those awesome omega-3s, which we know helps keep your brain nice and healthy. So mix up the meat party with some seafood once in a while. In fact, experts recommend that you have at least three servings of salmon (or some type of seafood) per week. Pretty awesome if you ask us because salmon is delicious and is super quick to prepare. Stay tuned for a few awesome salmon recipes.

Make sure you season your meat! Human beings need salt in our systems. Contrary to popular belief, salt is not the demon that science has made it out to be. Salt is absolutely necessary for us to function; in fact, one of the downsides to people doing the Keto diet is the "keto flu", which happens when people's electrolytes get all out of whack. How does that happen? They're not eating enough salt! So make sure you salt and season your food. Also, use other spices – spices have a plethora of health benefits and can help you get other nutrients that you need.

Finally, make sure you are drinking bone broth or something with collagen in it. Collagen isn't just that stuff that people inject into their faces so that they don't look like they have wrinkles. Collagen is an essential connective tissue in your body that also helps to cushion your joints and, well, definitely help you maintain that youthful look.

Do I do this for the rest of my life?

This diet can be followed for the rest of your life if you find that it's something that suits you.

So that's pretty much it, friends! Very few rules to follow and you can totally change your life. Get some good habits under your belt, buy some different groceries, get out and exercise – that's all you really have to do!

Chapter 4: What to Eat And What To Avoid

Approved foods:

- Beef
- Lamb
- Pork
- Chicken

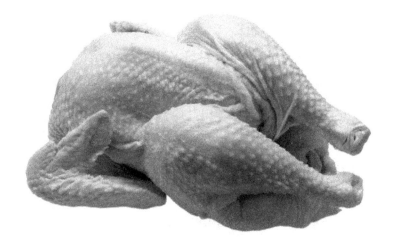

- Fish – salmon, whitefish, tilapia, trout, mackerel, sardines, crab, lobster, shrimp, scallops
- Ribeye
- Sirloin
- Strip steaks
- Chuck roast

- Prime rib
- Brisket
- Ground beef
- Liver
- Heart
- Kidneys
- Chicken wings
- Chicken thighs
- Chicken drumsticks
- Chicken breast
- Duck breast
- Duck wings
- Duck legs
- Duck confit (especially good because of its high fat content.)
- Eggs

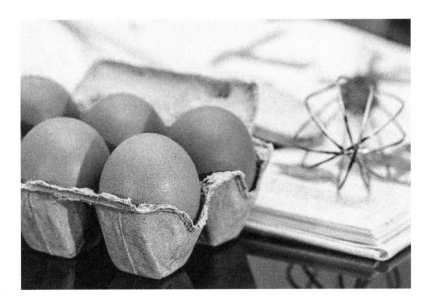

- Cheese
- Milk
- Cream
- Butter

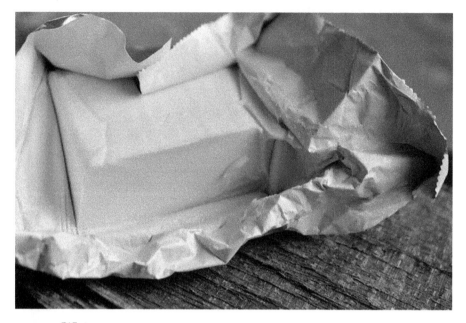

- Water
- Coffee
- Teas

Foods to Avoid:

- Fruits
- Vegetables
- Soda
- Alcohol
- Sweeteners

- Sugar
- Desserts
- Anything that is not meat or meat-related

*You should also avoid deli meats, as they tend to include fillers that contain carbohydrates

Here we are going to give you some nutritional facts about the foods that are allowed on this diet. We are not going to give you the nutrition fats for every single one of the allowed foods, but we will cover a lot of the heavy hitters.

Nutrition information for beef (ground):

Per 3 oz:

Calories	213
Fat	13 g
Cholesterol	77 mg
Total carbs	0 g
Protein	22 g
Vitamin B12	36% of Daily Value
Iron	12% of Daily Value
Vitamin B-6	4% of Daily Value

Nutrition information lamb (ground and otherwise):

Per 3oz:

Calories	250
Fat	18 g
Cholesterol	82 mg
Total carbs	0 g
Protein	21 g
Vitamin B12	36% of Daily Value
Iron	8% of Daily Value
Vitamin B-6	5% of Daily Value

Nutrition information pork (tenderloin):

Per 3oz:

Calories	122
Fat	3 g
Cholesterol	62 mg
Total carbs	0 g
Protein	22 g
Vitamin B12	28% of Daily Value
Iron	5% of Daily Value

Vitamin B-6	30% of Daily Value

Nutrition information salmon (fillet):

Per 3oz:

Calories	177
Fat	11 g
Cholesterol	47 mg
Total carbs	0 g
Protein	17 g
Vitamin B12	45% of Daily Value
Iron	1% of Daily Value
Vitamin B-6	25% of Daily Value

Nutrition information chicken breast (boneless and skinless):

Per 3oz:

Calories	165
Fat	3.6 g
Cholesterol	85 mg
Total carbs	0 g

Protein	31 g
Vitamin B12	5% of Daily Value
Iron	5% of Daily Value
Vitamin B-6	30% of Daily Value

Nutrition information duck breast:

Per 3oz:

Calories	337
Fat	28 g
Cholesterol	84 mg
Total carbs	0 g
Protein	19 g
Vitamin B12	5% of Daily Value
Iron	15% of Daily Value
Vitamin B-6	10% of Daily Value

Nutrition information scallops:

Per 3oz:

Calories	90
Fat	.5 g
Cholesterol	35 mg
Total carbs	5 g
Protein	17 g
Vitamin B12	0% of Daily Value
Iron	2% of Daily Value
Vitamin B-6	0% of Daily Value

Nutrition information chicken livers:

Per 3oz:

Calories	116
Fat	4.8 g
Cholesterol	77 mg
Total carbs	0 g
Protein	22 g
Vitamin B12	276% of Daily Value
Iron	49.9% of Daily Value

Vitamin B-6	42.7% of Daily Value

Nutrition information Eggs:

Per 1 egg:

Calories	78
Fat	5 g
Cholesterol	187 mg
Total carbs	0.6 g
Protein	6 g
Vitamin B12	10% of Daily Value
Iron	3% of Daily Value
Vitamin B-6	5% of Daily Value

As I said, this is not an exhaustive list of nutrition information for every allowable food on this diet. That being said, we think this a pretty good foundation for you to get started and do your own research. You will see pretty easily that animal protein can provide much more than just lots of healthy fats and a good amount of protein. It is a good source of vitamins and minerals as well. Especially once you begin to add in spices and seasonings. It will become a way for you to reclaim your health, one day at a time.

Chapter 5: Pros And Cons Of The Carnivore Diet

Allow me to begin first by stating that I am not a medical professional. I am not a doctor, in any sense of the word. So before you begin any kind of diet or exercise program, please consult the expert advice of a physician. There is a reason why they go to school for 8+ years and have to pass all sorts of exams and state boards – they need to know their stuff so that they can give sound advice.

Okay, now that being said, let us dive a little deeper into The Carnivore Diet by examining its pros and cons. Everything has pros and cons – nothing is perfect. They still haven't discovered a magic pill to weightloss with zero side effects and 100% guaranteed results. So anything you try will have its downsides. The key is to pick a diet and a lifestyle with as few downsides as possible. We happen to think that the Carnivore Diet is one example of a diet and lifestyle with very few downsides.

<u>Pros:</u>

The biggest pro of this particular diet is its effect on losing fat quickly. People who have tried this diet for 30-90 days have reported incredible weight loss. As with any diet, the first several pounds are going to be water weight as your body adjusts to a new way of eating. However, after that initial water weight drop, your body begins to use its fuel more efficiently and begins to burn away the excess fat that was stored from years of eating carbohydrates. Carbohydrates are sugars, plain and simple. Sugars get stored in the body as excess fat when we do not use enough energy to burn it off.

You can eliminate that problem by eliminating the sugars that you consume in the form of carbohydrates. By going on an all protein and high fat diet, you are automatically eliminating sugar from your diet. Studies have shown that eliminating sugar from your diet has beneficial effects not just on your waistline, but also in terms of thought clarity and even depression. They call carbohydrates comfort food, but in reality, they may be making some of your depression symptoms worse. Switching to a high protein and higher fat diet may help eliminate some of those symptoms.

A diet that is high in protein and fat is also going to end up giving you all of the micronutrients you need, without all the excess sugars that you don't need. Most people think that in order to get at all the itty bitty micronutrients that we humans need in order to function, you have to eat plants. Now, there are studies that show that plants and the foods derived from plants do contain these micronutrients. However, it has not been shown yet that those micronutrients are easily available for humans to absorb and use.

So what does this mean? It means that the micronutrients in plants are not necessarily bioavailable. When humans eat and digest plants, those plants need to be converted by the human body into the nutrients that we need in order to survive. More often than not, those nutrients get lost in the conversion process and we just need to keep eating more and more plants (more and more carbohydrates) in order to get the proper amounts of these micronutrients. That is just wildly inefficient and not to mention expensive.

Studies have shown that meat has much more bioavailability than plants and plant-related foods. This means that when we eat meat and fats, we are able to more easily absorb the nutrients that are contained within the meat. Meat, after all, was once a creature that feasted on plant matter and those nutrients that the creatures have absorbed now is in their flesh. So, when we eat meat, we are able to access the nutrients that were stored in their flesh over their lives.

That is why it is important (and we will get into this later on in the book) for you to choose meats and fats that are the highest quality that you can get. When you get grass fed beef, for example, you are eating beef that has literally been infused with the nutrients found in plant matter, but in a form that is much easier for you, a human, to digest and absorb. In fact, some of the most necessary micronutrients for human function are creatine, carnosine, and vitamin B12, all of which exist in meat. Without those essential micronutrients, you would be seriously unhealthy.

Cons:

As I mentioned before, there can be no upside without a downside. Yes, there are going to be a few things that are not perfect about the carnivore diet, and we will touch on each of them briefly here.

First, you are going to face some boredom. Eating meat and only meat will get repetitive after a while, unless you're the kind of person who really and truly thrives on routine. That's why, later on in this book, we are going to provide you with 30 different recipe ideas: 10 for breakfast, 10 for dinner, and 10 for dessert. Because yes, when you are going through something like a major lifestyle change, if you don't have some semblance of what you love and enjoy eating, you will snap, binge, and then have to start all over from square one. Nobody wants that.

Another possible downside is if you a person who is prone to high blood pressure or who smokes and just generally leads an unhealthy lifestyle, you are going to want to one, talk to your doctor about getting your blood pressure under control and see if you can bring it under control and if it is safe for you to go on this diet. And if you are a smoker or someone who just lives an unhealthy lifestyle, just know that starting to eat bacon every day is not going to solve your problems. You are going to need to put in work to make sure that this is a lifestyle overhaul, not just a band-aid on a bigger problem in your life.

In later chapters, we will discuss the motivations for going on this diet and help you outline what you hope to achieve by becoming carnivorous. Read on!

Chapter 6: Differences Between The Carnivore Diet, Keto, And The Paleo Diet

Believe it or not, there are very big differences between these diets, even though they have the same basic principle: do not eat processed foods! The idea of these diets is to get us to a point where we were before all of these processed foods started showing up in our diets. Humans were a good deal healthier before we exposed ourselves to pesticides, preservatives, and a host of other chemicals that are in our food today. But this particular section is going to focus on the differences so that you can navigate your way between these diets with ease.

The Paleo Diet

This is probably one of the most recognized diets the world over. Made famous by CrossFit and the subject of blogs all across the internet, this diet has more words devoted to it than you can possibly imagine. Its appeal is that it is easy to follow, fun to experiment with, and has shown itself to have long-lasting benefits to those who follow it.

The Paleo diet focuses on whole, nutritionally dense foods that are not processed. It is heavy on meat and vegetables and also dials in on healthy fats. One of the biggest draws of the Paleo diet is the fact that you are able to get in a lot of good flavors with your recipes because you can add in so many different fats. Coconut oil and grass-fed ghee are two of the favorite fats on the Paleo diet and for good reason. Coconut oil has many health benefits and if you get refined coconut oil, you can use it in any recipe without it tasting like the inside of a coconut. Ghee, or clarified butter, is a great addition because it has all the flavor of butter without the gut-irritating milk solids.

But I think we are getting a little ahead of ourselves here. So, what's allowed on the Paleo diet? Meat, vegetables, a little fruit, and healthy fats like coconut oil, olive oil, and ghee. Flavorings like coconut aminos and spices are also welcomed on this diet. (There are alternatives to this diet called AIP, or autoimmune protocol, which eliminate certain vegetables and spices, but we won't concern ourselves with the AIP in this section of the book. Look to the section "Who is the Carnivore Diet For?" for further explanation of the autoimmune protocol.)

Foods to be avoided on the Paleo diet is anything that comes in a package or a box, artificial sweeteners, vegetable oils (they have some carcinogenic qualities, and also don't really taste very good), grains, legumes, nuts, and dairy. The reason the diet eliminates processed foods is fairly obvious – they aren't good for you! While I can't deny that a bag of Doritos can be relatively satisfying after a stressful day at work, they are also not really...well, food.

But what about dairy? I hear you, I do, but for a lot of people, dairy is a gut irritant that they could easily do without. In fact, you may not realize it, but you may have a dairy intolerance. Just because you don't get violently ill after eating dairy doesn't mean that you're not lactose intolerant. Do you have joint pain? Or problems with your skin? Or maybe chronic constipation? Maybe take a look at your dairy consumption and see if you can connect any dots. You would be surprised at what you would find.

Also, I hope you aren't surprised when I tell you that grains and legumes are also known inflammatory substances. Most people, if not everyone in the entire world, are aware of celiac disease. This means that people are allergic to gluten, which is a protein formed when wheat and water mix together. It's a little more complicated than that, but hey – I'm not a chemist. The point is gluten can make people get very sick and have reactions from severe vomiting and stomach bloating to more mild symptoms like achy joints and lowered immune systems.

Legumes are not a trigger for celiac disease, but they do irritate the gut and the digestive tract. I'm sure you are aware of the effect beans have on the digestive tract. This is because they are too hard for the body to digest effectively – which means that there also isn't much nutrition that is being absorbed when we eat these little kidney-shaped things.

The Paleo diet also has other variations for people to adapt to their lifestyles. One that I would like to spend a moment talking about is the Autoimmune Protocol, or the AIP version of the Paleo diet. As you may be aware since you are reading a book about a diet, quite a few people (several million) suffer from autoimmune diseases. These are diseases in which the immune system attacks the body. It often results in joint pain, inflamed digestive tract, poor immune health, weight gain, and a host of other issues.

Fed up with the medical community, people who have these diseases often turn to a more holistic way of healing their afflictions. One such way is through their diet. These diets focus on eliminating foods that are known to inflame the body. So they are very restrictive, but people have reported excellent results after only a few months of following these protocols. One such protocol is the autoimmune protocol version of the Paleo diet. It eliminates things like nightshade vegetables, certain spices, and even egg whites. (Who knew egg whites were inflammatory, right? I know I didn't before I started researching these different diets.)

Personally, I suffer from Hashimoto's Disease. Basically, this means that not only does my thyroid not produce enough of its hormone, but I also have a hard time losing weight, my immune system generally stinks, and my joints are almost always inflamed. But that's what started my search for a way to heal my body that wasn't just pills. My medication from my doctor works, and I trust what my doctor says, but I needed to feel better. So I was researching different ways to heal autoimmune diseases and the autoimmune protocol version of the Paleo diet popped up. As did the ketogenic and carnivore diets, which we will cover next!

Macro and Micronutrients:

In case you did not notice by the fact that I am writing a diet book, I am kind of a nerd about this kind of stuff. Food and its chemical breakdown is absolutely fascinating to me. The processes that our bodies use to break down, absorb, and then use the food that we eat are endlessly interesting to me. To that end, I have devoted years of my life to researching diets, exercise, and the ways in which we calculate our nutrient needs.

So let us talk for just a minute about how to calculate our macros. This will help you lose weight no matter what diet you are on. As long as your macros are being met, you can generally eat what you like. Of course, these macronutrients are not going to be as important when you are on the carnivore diet, because, well, your food options are generally much less open. But for the sake of educating and for the sake of giving you as much information as you need in order to be successful in weight management over the course of your life, we are going to explain how to calculate your macros.

First, you need to figure out how many calories you burn while simply resting. This formula will differ for men and women, but they are as follows:

Men: 10 x Weight(in kg) + 6.25 x height (in cm) − 5 x age(years) +5 = BMR

Women: 10 x Weight(in kg) + 6.25 x height (in cm) − 5 x age(years) -161 = BMR

BMR means your basal metabolic rate, or how many calories you burn while sitting on the couch, binge-watching the latest show on Netflix.

Next, you need to figure out how much energy you expend on a normal day, which includes getting up, moving around, and also working out, if you are that kind of person. You are going to take your BMR and multiply it by a scalable variant that matches your activity level. If you are very active, you are going to multiply your BMR by 1.75. If you are moderately active, multiply your BMR by 1.55. If you experience light activity, then multiply your BMR by 1.375. And then if you are a total couch potato (no judgment – everyone has to start somewhere), multiply your BMR by 1.2.

This will give you how many calories you would need to eat just to maintain your weight. To lose weight, you will need to cut those total daily calories by 500 each day to lose 1 pound of body fat. To gain, add in an extra five hundred calories each day. Now for the super fun math part.

So, you may not know this, but 1 gram of protein is "worth" four calories. One gram of carbohydrates is worth four calories as well. 1 gram of fat has nine calories. Let us use protein first. To calculate your daily protein intake, simply multiply .825 by your body weight. This will give you how many grams of protein you will need to eat each day. So if you weight 200 pounds, you need roughly 165 grams of protein each day.

Next, let us talk a little about fat. Contrary to popular belief about weight loss, fat is your friend. Fat helps you feel fuller longer and it also contains many vital nutrients that your body needs. Our bodies need fat in order to run properly. There have been many studies and world examples that show that when people do not have a high enough body fat percentage, their health takes a severe decline. Women can often lose their menstrual periods and even become infertile. Both men and women are more susceptible to disease when their body fat percentages are too low. So, what I am saying here is that fat is important and you will want to include it in your diet no matter what particular diet plan you may be following.

So, let's say you allocate 25% of your calories to your fat intake. Simply multiply your calories that you will be eating by .25. Then divide that number by nine, which are the calories per gram that fat has. Then, eat that many grams of fat per day.

Then figuring out how many calories are left and dedicate those calories to carbohydrates. Because even though I am writing a book about the carnivore diet, I will not deny that I enjoy carbohydrates. I think everyone does, really. And like I have said in other parts of this book, I will not say that this is a diet that you will follow for the rest of your life. The carnivore diet is a great way to jump-start weight loss, but it does not have to be the diet you follow for the rest of your life. And that's why I wanted to give you a breakdown of how to find your macros. That way, should you decide to follow other methods of dieting when you feel like moving on from the carnivore diet.

We just want you to succeed at being the best version of yourself that you can possibly be. That is why we wrote this book. We believe that by putting out accurate information and giving people as much of a fighting chance against metabolic diseases as we can, then we are doing our job. We want you to be happy and healthy, no matter what. That's why we dedicated all the hours into this book and into the recipes and explanations – we believe that humanity is in need of good information about diet and exercise. So, with that being said, let us move on to moving on to a conclusion about the Paleo diet and start talking about the Keto diet and the Carnivore diet.

The really awesome thing is that the Paleo diet can be adapted to your particular nutrient needs. Without delving into a huge explanation, each person has unique calorie and macro and micronutrient needs. So, broadly speaking, each

But to sum it up, the AIP and Paleo diets can be a good starting point for people looking to overhaul their lives their diets. It is a good stepping-stone to ease yourself into a new way of eating and living so that you can decide oif a more restrictive way of eating is something you need.

The Ketogenic Diet

The Ketogenic (or Keto) diet takes the paleo diet a little further. This diet focuses on high fat, just enough protein, and very low in carbohydrates. The keto diet is based on the principle that if you are able to get enough fat into your diet and lower your carbohydrate intake enough, you can convince your body to use fat, your own body fat, as fuel.

Thus, it follows that as your body gets more and more efficient at burning fat as fuel, you will continue to lose body fat, gain muscle, and just be a fat burning machine with an epic six pack and great overall health. This is based on more than just theories, by the way. The keto diet has actually been around since 1923 when it was first used to first help people with epilepsy. So as annoyed as you may be with everyone on your Facebook newsfeed who is losing their minds over Keto, instead of being annoyed at them for all their spam, instead, feel sorry for them because they are just so darn late to the party. Since then, there have been several iterations of the keto diet, which have helped to address everything from epilepsy to diabetes.

The Science

Let's geek out for a minute about the science behind the ketogenic diet. I am, unashamedly, fascinated by the science here. So, we all know that the food we eat gets broken down by our bodies and then the nutrients that are released are absorbed and put to use. And it is obvious at this point that it matters what kind of fuel we put into our bodies. When we put garbage into the gas tank, we get garbage. And when we put extra special engine cleaning fuel into the tank, our Honda Civic suddenly feels like a Ferrari.

The keto diet is focused on turning our own body fat into the fuel for that Ferrari. So, when we reduce our carbohydrate consumption to epic lows and instead consume fat, we can put our body in a certain state called ketosis. Ketosis is a state our body enters when it is deprived of carbohydrates and turns to burning fat to maintain homeostasis. Pretty awesome, right?

That's because it is. Eventually, your body burns enough of your body fat to help you maintain a healthy weight and you can stop constantly worrying about that number on the scale. But of course, I need you to understand that I am not a doctor. I cannot replace the advice of medical professionals who are going to tell you what is best for you and your health. All I can do is give you enough information to make informed decisions and then eventually talk to your doctor about your decisions.

The Rules

Okay, so like I said, this diet really cuts back on the carbs and there are several iterations of the keto diet, just like there are iterations of the paleo diet. The original form of the keto diet, the one formed back in 1923, has the following macronutrient breakdown: 75% fat, 20% protein, and the rest is carbohydrates. This is the strictest version of the diet and also the one that has the most scientific backup.

Another iteration of the diet is a version where you cycle days on and off of higher and lower carbs. So, for example, if you were exercising particularly hard on Monday, maybe make that one of your higher carb days. If you are going to be skipping the gym and just working at your desk on Tuesday, then go ahead an make that a strict ketogenic day. See what I'm driving there? This particular version of the diet allows you to adjust your carbohydrate intake as your activity levels and lifestyle indicate.

Another way to lead a ketogenic lifestyle is to focus on more protein and more moderate fat than just the standard keto diet. This is just a step below the carnivore diet. (See, there is a method to my madness here.) Here, your diet is 60% fat, 35% protein, and then the rest is carbohydrate.

Now on to more nitty gritty facts. On the keto diet, again, you are trying to focus on whole, nutritionally dense foods. Yes, there are about a million products out there that are aimed at keto diet followers, but you do not need to spend your money on all of these powders, mixes, and bars. You can just go shopping at your regular grocery store, buy whole foods, and save yourself a whole lot of money. In fact, we have a whole section of this book dedicated to showing you how to save money at the grocery store when you are shopping for a higher protein and higher fat diet.

So remember, when you are following the keto diet, you are going to avoid packaged foods and foods that are high in carbohydrates. It is a little more forgiving than the paleo diet, in that you can still eat grains and dairy if they fit into your macros, but it is stricter in the sense that your carbohydrate consumption is much more restricted.

The Carnivore Diet

Okay, so now the section of this chapter that you all have ben waiting for. The carnivore diet! So here we are just going to give a brief overview of what makes the carnivore diet different and what separates it from these other diets that focus on heavy consumption of protein and fat.

So remember how I said that the paleo diet was a good starting point for getting your feet wet in regards to changing up your diet and lifestyle? The keto diet is the next step down the stricter path and the carnivore diet is about as strict as it gets in regards to diets that focus on high fat and high protein. The carnivore diet eschews any carbohydrates and focuses entirely on animal protein and fat. It relies on the principle of the keto diet that if you focus on fats and protein, your body will go into ketosis and use fat as its main source of fuel instead of carbohydrates. What this means is that your body fat will become fuel.

So while this is a diet that focuses heavily on fats and proteins, just like the paleo and keto diets, where it differs is in its execution. Here, you just focus on eating high quality animal proteins and fats. So while it is more restrictive, it is also much simpler. In other sections of the book, we will discuss foods to be eaten and foods to avoid. We will also discuss how to buy all of this high quality meat without breaking your bank.

Now you know! You know the difference between these three very popular diets. We hope that this portion of the book was helpful to you and will inform your decision about which diet plan to follow for yourself. Obviously, this is a book about the carnivore diet, but we want you to make a decision that will help make you the healthiest version of yourself.

Chapter 7: Who Is The Carnivore Diet For?

I could probably just end this chapter at the beginning and say that this diet is for everyone. But I don't really want to make such a general statement. While I do believe that this diet is one that can help most people, I am going to spend this section talking about diet culture, why the word 'diet' can be harmful to some people, why meat has been vilified for so long, and why it is important to do your research before you commit to a lifestyle and a way of eating.

Diet Culture

I could honestly write an entire book about diet culture and what that all means. But, alas, I am limited to a chapter. So I am going to talk to you about why diet culture is actually a thing and also how it can be incredibly harmful to people who are in it.

If you spend any time online, whether on Facebook or on Instagram, you are likely going to see ad after ad for diet pills, health coaches, and before and after photos of people who have miraculously lost an entire fifth grader in just six weeks. Diet culture is in the commercials we watch and the food we buy and the pop ups that are on our websites. It is unfortunate, but we are fed a constant barrage of information telling us that we are never going to be happy until we lose those last five pesky pounds.

What they don't tell you is that each person is different. Yes, one person can get a six-pack while eating Doritos and just working out all of the time. Another must weigh each and every gram of food and program their workouts down to the moment. One approach is not necessarily better than the other. Though please do not think that I am advocating for you to just eat Doritos and hope that you can work it off in the gym.

Each of those people have different caloric needs, different micronutrient needs, different needs when it comes to programming workouts. And each of those people have different things that will make them happy. Maybe a six-pack will make them happy. Or having arms like Chris Hemsworth. Or a waist like Anna Kendrick. Who knows. What I do know is that not everybody wants those things and not everybody needs those things to be happy.

I am not here to be your therapist or to tell you exactly what you do need to make you happy. What I am here to say is that if you are unhappy with your life and you think that all you need is just to lose some weight...you will never actually be happy. You will continue to pick apart your appearance and your performance until you just can't stand it any more. Before you start down a weight loss journey, it helps to be really crystal clear about your intentions.

I personally started my own weight loss journey for the wrong reasons. I wanted to lose weight because I was unhappy and because I thought that if I lost my excess weight, then that would be the key to my happiness. So I tried everything I could to lose weight, short of going under the knife. I tried pills, I starved and binged, I tried every insane diet under the sun that I thought could help me lose weight quickly. I didn't care about losing it safely or about making sure that I didn't do more harm than good to my body or my mind. I just wanted to lose the weight.

So I did. I lost an enormous amount of weight in an extremely unhealthy way. I damaged my mind and body in a quest to make myself 'happy'. And all I did was make myself even more miserable. So you know what happened next? I gained half of the weight back. There was no physical way I could continue the way I was and live. So I chose to live and rebuild. That of course meant that some of the weight was going to come back. That was inevitable.

But I started to do the actual hard work. I went to therapy. I got a nutritionist. I also got a personal trainer. I began to learn things about myself and about my body that I had ignored for years. Turns out, I actually really like food. Turns out I am also really good at lifting heavy stuff. So I finally figured out a way to marry those two sides of my personality and now I am finally both happy and healthy.

So before we go to the next section in this chapter, I want you to understand that before you embark on any sort of diet and exercise plan, it is imperative that you don't just talk to a medical doctor, but that you also talk to yourself. Figure out your true motivations and reasons for wanting to lose weight. And then promise yourself that you are going to do this in a safe and healthy manner.

So what's wrong with the word 'diet'?

Again, this is another subject that I could write an entire book about. But I promise that I will keep this in similar length to the previous section about diet culture. But the word diet can be so incredibly harmful, especially to people who have an eating disorder. It reinforces the idea that in order for them to have any semblance of "order", they need to follow certain strict rules for living and eating.

This word has taken on such a misconstrued meaning – anything can be a diet. Eating just Fritos and ding-dongs is a diet. A diet is just what you eat, nothing more and nothing less. A diet does not have to mean a restrictive way of eating. A diet is simply comprised of whatever it is you eat – whether that be a powerlifter's diet of force feeding meals in order to gain mass or a bikini competitor's prep meal schedule. So don't think that just because this is a 'diet', you are restricting yourself. The whole idea behind this way of eating is that you are actually rewarding yourself and treating your body with love and care.

If you feel, though, that you are eating this way to punish yourself for eating "badly" before or because you feel like if you just start eating a lot of steak you'll suddenly love yourself, maybe take a minute and really try to identify the reasons behind you revamping your life and eating habits. Because that's what this is, really. It's just a way to revamp your eating habits and start to gain back health and lose some excess fat.

This is not a way to discover inner happiness or fix something that is broken in your life. This is a way to gain health - that is all. Yes, when you are healthier you are happier. This is indisputable. But a new diet is not going to all of a sudden make you love yourself or take the place of a therapist if you need one. I know that I have said this in probably a million different ways, but it is just so important. Before you start on a diet, even this one, make sure your intentions and goals are crystal-clear. Then go buy some steak.

Okay, but really, who is the carnivore diet for?

If you have an underlying health problem, then you should probably talk to your doctor before you begin any kind of diet and exercise program. Scratch that – *definitely* talk to your doctor or other health care professional before beginning any kind of diet and exercise routine. As I said, all of my research and reading and experimenting still cannot and should not replace a medical degree. Those are some pretty smart folks. Plus, your doctor will actually know you and your medical history, which is invaluable when recommending lifestyle changes.

This diet is for people who have tried so many different diets and yet still have stubborn weight that just won't leave. Kind of like that ex-boyfriend who left his dog in your apartment, you just can't keep it from coming back. Well, time to say goodbye. If you are absolutely fed up with complicated diets, counting calories, and just the general amount of effort that tends to go into these fancy diets nowadays, then the carnivore diet is for you.

I don't know about you, but I genuinely hate counting calories. Who wants to break out a calculator and a scale every time they are hungry and want to have a meal? I get far too angry when that happens and usually just end up eating whatever I wanted anyway because by the time I was done figuring out the calorie count and whether the meal fit into my macros, I was just too hungry to care any more. I also have a small son, so you try to keep a two-year old away from sharp objects in the kitchen and the zillion other things in a house that is designed to kill them while also trying to make a food that perfectly fits into your macros. Go ahead. I'll wait.

... Back yet? Okay, so you see my point, right? Doing things that way can work for some people. I, in fact, know several people who have used the macro counting and food prep system for years to great effect. I am just not that organized when it comes to my personal life. I really am not. Professionally, I am a star – deadlines are always met, initiative is taken, and I'm always the first one in the office. And when it comes to my son, I'm always on top of things. Doctor's appointments are kept, he's signed up for sports, and his laundry is always done and freshly folded.

But as for me, personally, I just don't have the energy to sit down with a scale, calculator, and Tupperware to make sure that each meal is picture perfect. I did it once, for a week. I thought I was going to lose my mind. And then I came upon the carnivore diet. Just eat meat and fats and make sure they are coming from happy and healthy animals. That's it! No weird food prep methods, no expensive supplements, and no crazy rules I had to follow. Awesome.

So if you are like me and just need a little simplicity in your life, then this is the diet for you. Of course, not everyone who follows this diet is a single mom of a toddler who is trying to keep at least five different plates spinning at one time. This is also a great diet for strength athletes who are looking to increase their muscle tone. We all know that protein builds muscle. So, what's going to happen when you eat a ton more protein? You are going to build muscle! Also, because you are introducing lots of healthy fats to the party, you are also going to help protect yourself from lots of different communicable diseases, which will inevitably help your athletic performance. A track athlete is not going to win any meets if they can't breathe out of their nose due to a sinus infection.

Do you remember the television show 'Parks and Rec'? With Amy Poehler and Chris Pratt before he got hot? It was a great show. Rob Lowe had a recurring spot on the show as "Chris", a government bureaucrat who exercised almost every single minute of the day. He was also relentlessly and annoyingly positive, but we are going to focus on the exercise portion of this particular anecdote here. So, as I said, he was obsessed with eating healthy and exercising. But during one episode, a severe flu hits the town.

Desperate and sweaty, he shows up to the hospital and is crying out that his body is a microchip – a single grain of sand can upset the whole balance of the microchip. His body is like a microchip because his body fat percentage is around 5%. This leaves him vulnerable to things like the flu. Without a good supply of fat, our bodies are left defenseless to things like colds and the flu. Don't be like a microchip – don't let a silly cold be the thing that derails you, all because you wanted to have a super low body fat percentage.

But I digress. (I just really, really love that show.) This is a diet for people who aren't afraid of fat and who aren't afraid to eat a lot of protein to keep their body running like a well-oiled machine. It's for people who need an uncomplicated way to lose and keep off the weight without rules and supplements. It is for people who want to eat real food and get satisfaction from their meals.

Speaking of satisfaction and meals, in our next chapter, we are going to talk about how to save money when you are shopping for all this meat!

Chapter 8: Carnivore Diet Tips for Success

Dealing with the Keto Flu

Perhaps the worst part of switching to the Carnivore Diet is that entering ketosis is more difficult for the body than simply cutting out most of your carbs for a few days. This is due to the fact that the Standard American Diet is so full of carbs that your body has likely never developed the tools it needs to generate fuel from fat in the most efficient ways possible. As such, it is naturally going to take at least a week for your body to truly get with the program and generate the level of fuel you need to operate as effectively as possible. This period between when you give up carbs and when your body starts producing and using ketones at maximum capacity is known as the keto flu and it is almost certainly going to be rough going.

For starters, you will notice a severe drop in your energy levels along with the other sorts of flu symptoms you would expect. While this week is going to be difficult to handle, it is important to keep in mind that it is a vital part of the process which is only occurring because of your existing reliance on carbs. If you want your body to fuel itself in a more effective fashion then this is the only way.

The most important thing to remember during this time is that you cannot, under any circumstances, give in and dramatically increase your carb intake, not even once. If you do give in to your cravings then you will undo all of your hard work in an instant as your body will go back to fueling itself with carbs which means you will need to wait until they are all out of your system before you can start all over again. Stay strong and remember the keto flu almost never lasts more than a week.

During the transition, you may find some relief if you add a fourth meal to your diet sometime between lunch and dinner. If this doesn't seem to make things better, just remember that each time you feel a pang of carb-based hunger it is just another step towards ketosis. During this timeframe, you are going to want to limit yourself to no more than 15 net grams of carbs per day. Net carbs can be determined by taking the number of carbs that you consume in a day and subtract from that the amount of fiber you consume in the same period.

You may find it helpful to test yourself throughout this process to ensure you are moving in the right direction. What you will be testing yourself for is a substance called acetone which is produced when a ketone is broken down to generate energy. You can purchase either blood or urine tests that will indicate your current ketone level which should be somewhere between .5 when you start ketosis and 3 when your body gets used to the process. You can also determine if you are in the ketogenic state if your breath begins to smell like a slightly rotten apple and tastes slightly metallic. If, when testing yourself, you find that your ketone level rises above 3 then you are going to want to increase the number of calories you are consuming per day as your body is not getting enough of the calories it needs to function at peak effectiveness.

Another great way to make it through the transition is through the use of what are known as fat bombs. After you have removed practically all of the carbohydrates from your diet you are likely going to feel a carbohydrate-sized hole in your diet, especially when it comes to grabbing a quick snack or looking to something to provide a quick burst of energy which is where the fat bomb comes into play. A fat bomb is a quick to eat snack that can be either sweet or savory and is full of healthy fats from things like butter, coconut oil, seeds and nuts which means they are often 80 or 90 percent healthy fat per serving.

Not only will the energy in these snacks get you up and moving, the healthy fats will fill you up and satiate you until your next proper meal rolls around. Even better, it will do both of these things in a way that is much more effective than the carbohydrate filled fashion to which you are likely already accustomed to. This means they are the perfect choice if you are planning on going to the gym or know you won't have time to fix yourself a healthy dinner until later than normal. What's more, they will help you to get your daily allotment of fats in each day which is going to be more difficult some days than you might expect.

While fat bombs can be a quick, easy and, most importantly, healthy option to round out your diet, that doesn't mean they shouldn't still be consumed in moderation, especially at first. It is important to keep in mind that your body might have an initially poor reaction to so much fat, healthy or no, so you will want to introduce all your new dietary regulars over a period of a week or so to ensure that your body doesn't have any other major dietary concerns to consider while it is making the difficult transition to ketosis.

Saving Money

One of the biggest misconceptions about following this particular diet is that you are going to end up in debt just to put food on the table. That is most certainly not the case. I am going to spend this chapter talking to you about how you can save some money while also improving your health.

First, on this diet, you do not need to waste your money on supplements, powders, or packaged bars to make your meals complete. I cannot even tell you many billions of dollars are spent each year on health "supplements" that have about as much effectiveness as telling yourself that the water in your glass magically turns into vodka when it passes your lips. Trust me, I've tried. I am not magic. But you are also not wasting any money on protein powders or expensive protein bars.

This diet does not call for you to make protein shakes or eat protein bars, even though it is a diet that focuses almost exclusively on protein. The reason behind this is that our bodies do not effectively absorb the protein in those sorts of foods as easily as they do from regular meat. Not to mention that many, many protein powders on the market today contain additives that can really upset your stomach. And when I say upset your stomach, I mean make it swell up like a balloon and cause other...issues. So unless you want to waste your money on ground up protein that's just going to cause you to have incredible amounts of gastrointestinal distress, then I suggest you skip them altogether and follow the rules outlined here in this diet.

Okay, so the first rule of saving money when you are shopping on this diet is to buy in bulk. Before you go shopping, clear out your refrigerator and freezer of everything that does not follow the plan or that will trip you up while you adjust to this new way of eating and living. Because you are going to be buying up meat in bulk, which means you are going to need to store things for a while. Your freezer is going to be your friend.

When you buy in bulk, you are able to save a lot of money. For example, did you know that you can buy filet mignon in a bulk form and then cut it to size yourself? Well, you can. And it's fabulous. A quick Google search or a few dollars on iTunes will get you 'Tender is the Loin 1'. This is not a weird video about meat fetishists or something like that. It is an episode of the absolutely amazing show 'Good Eats' hosted by the incredibly talented Mr. Alton Brown.

I'm sure you have heard of Mr. Brown, considering he is now the star of several food-related shows and even has a traveling tour around the United States. He dedicated several episodes of his now-famous television show to the wonderful cut of beef known as the filet mignon. But this particular episode walks you through how to pick out a perfect beef tenderloin and then break it down into its various parts. It is so much more budget-conscious (not to mention delicious) to buy an entire tenderloin and then break it down into steaks by yourself. That way you can freeze what you are not ready to eat and get the benefit of stretching out that much meat over several months.

So go download that episode, take some notes, and then head out to buy yourself a nice big tenderloin. I promise that you will not regret it. I happen to think that you will end up becoming a fan of 'Good Eats' for life and you will thank the stars that you bought yourself a beef tenderloin and learned how to break it down yourself.

You also will want to scour your grocery store's circular for meat deals every week. In my particular town, we have a store called Acme. Yeah, just like the cartoons. Except that we don't get anvils dropped on our head when we enter the store, which I suppose is a bonus. But we do get amazing deals on meat every single week. Also, one week a year, we have "steak week", which is one magical week where there is a special meat sale. We can get seven pounds of meat for seven dollars. That is a pretty insane deal if you ask me. So my family and I load up on meat during that week and freeze what we don't eat. We then have meals for the rest of the year.

Another great tip to make your dollar stretch a little more when you switch to this eating plan is to make meals in a batch. This will also save you time because when you come home from a long day at work, you can just heat up something already prepared instead of taking the time to make a new meal. So why will making batch meals save you money? Well, consider this: how often do you find yourself shelling out money every day for lunch or breakfast? How often do you find yourself so tired and just *done* by the end of the day that you end up calling out for food or going to your local fast food place?

If you end up adding up all of this money that you're spending on food that other people cook, you will see that you spend thousands of dollars on food that you could have just cooked yourself. So when you make a batch meal, you are taking advantage of our first principle, which is to buy meat in bulk. You are also taking advantage of our second principle here, which is to save money by cooking your food yourself.

Also, remember what I was saying earlier about pesticides and chemicals and all kinds of additives that are in our food nowadays? Yeah, those things are bad, bad news. But guess what you get to avoid when you cook your own meals? Yeah! When you take cooking into your own hands, you are able to avoid putting in unnecessary chemicals into your food, which is a monumental step in making you a happier and healthier version of yourself.

A third tip is to buy the cheaper cuts. Yes, I know that I just talked your ear off about filet mignon, but people have been creating beautiful meals out of the cheap cuts for years. Cassoulet – that famous French dish that you would pay about $25 for in a restaurant? Cheap cuts! Hanger steak, the new buzzword on every food show imaginable? Cheap cut! The best ragu sauce you will ever taste? Yeah, made with pork neck bones. What does that mean? It's a cheap cut! Cheap cuts of meat can create things that you wouldn't imagine. So do me a favor. Go out and buy Julia Child's The Art of French Cooking and look through it. Find out the recipes that use the cheap cuts and adapt them for your own uses. Trust me when I say that it will change your life.

Anthony Bourdain also has a lot to say about cheap cuts of meat and has some good ideas on how to use them. I would recommend checking out his Les Halles cookbook (Les Halles was the restaurant he was cooking at before he got all famous.) It gives you details on how he used the cheaper cuts of meat at his restaurant and turned them into delicious dishes that his customers would beat down his door for. I also would recommend checking out his book 'Appetites', because while it may not have a lot of recipes for cheap cuts of meat, but it does have recipes that are uncomplicated and uses every day ingredients that you don't need to source from Amazon or a store where you pay $20 per ounce for herbs.

What will I do with all this money I'm going to save?

Now, I also want to tell you that saving all of this money by buying in bulk and making batch meals (with cheap cuts!) means that you can spend a little extra of that money by making sure that you are buying high quality meats and fats. I encourage you to follow some of the rules that I am going to outline below about how to make sure you are buying meats that are high quality and will help nourish your body beyond the factory farmed meats that most of us eat every day. I am going to talk about our three main land proteins – beef, pork, and chicken. I will also briefly cover salmon, because that is a fish most people are familiar with and are comfortable eating, buying, and preparing.

First, you need to make sure that the beef you are buying is grass-fed. Grass-fed beef has so many advantages to it that I could wax on and on about it. But here are some of the important things you need to know. Grass-fed beef will, most importantly, taste better than grain fed. Yes, it will taste different at first, since we are all so used to grain-fed beef. But I promise, once you make that transition, you will wonder how you ate grain-fed beef all of your life. Also, grass-fed beef has better marbling of fat throughout the meat. This means that the meat will be more tender and just fall apart after cooking. Nobody likes a tough cut of meat.

Grass-fed beef is also better for the planet. The amount of land that goes into raising enough grain for cattle to feed on is absolutely insane – that much land needs fertilizer, pesticides, and farming equipment. All of which help to emit CO_2. I don't need to tell you that is not good for the planet. Even if you don't 'believe' in climate change, you understand that wasting resources benefits no one. It is a waste of resources to use enormous tracts of land and waste farmers' time raising grain to feed cattle. Grass grows naturally and is also a crop that does not deplete the soil. It all makes sense – just eat the grass fed beef. You're already saving money by clipping coupons, buying in bulk, and getting the cheap cuts – so invest a little bit of what you're saving and buy the grass-fed stuff.

Okay, so now on to the pork. Numerous studies have shown that happy pigs mean better meat. I know that sounds sadistic, but it's true. When an animal is raised in a humane manner and given good food to eat, the meat that it produces is healthier and is free from all kinds of nasty hormones that are emitted by the animal's body when it lives in fear and filth. So what does this mean when it comes to pork? You need to look for animals that are raised on a farm by a farmer who actually cares about the animals he or she is raising. In all honesty, what will make the most sense as far as both saving money and making sure that you are getting the highest quality product that is going to fuel your Ferrari?

If you want a great example of this, I urge you to take a look at Michael Pollan's excellent documentary: "Cooked". You can watch it on Netflix and if you've ever watched Joss Whedon's 'Firefly', you'll know what I'm saying when I tell you that the pain of having the show end will stay with you for a while. You think that it's going to be just another cooking show and then your mind is just blown. This particular documentary covers the four basic elements – fire, water, earth, and air – and how they play into how we cook and eat. It talks about the rise of pesticides and preservatives in our food and how it has affected our health. I really wish I could spend more time telling you about this amazing documentary, but the biggest thing you can learn from this documentary is that you should buy your pork from local farmers. Call them up and reserve either a whole or half a pig – it will last you for months, possibly even a year. And you will be able to enjoy your meal that much more, knowing that not only are you supporting a local farmer, but you are also contributing to better welfare for these animals that provide our food.

I also would like to take a moment and talk about chicken. I will be bluntly honest with you – I hate chickens. I was chased and pecked by a flock of them when I was a child and have carried a grudge ever since. So I am not going to be one of those people you see on Facebook who is lovingly caressing a chicken. I prefer my chickens baked with a side of sweet potatoes, thank you. Now, as I have grown up, I have developed a little more empathy for my feathered friends. And I think you should, too.

We eat these creatures, yes. They are here to provide us with food. But that does not mean that we get to treat them with cruelty or disrespect. If anything, it means that we should honor those creatures who give their lives so that we may eat. And that means that we give them good food, a place to roam, and clean accommodations that protect them from the elements. Too often, chickens are kept in cages that are far too small, to the point where they cannot even walk or turn their heads. I would keep describing their living conditions, but it honestly disturbs me, so I will just say that factory farming is a process that needs to stop. When you go to buy chicken, make sure you are buying from a local farmer who lets their birds roam and eat a high quality vegetarian diet. This will be a little more expensive, but you are doing good things for the planet and for your community.

Finally, let's talk about farmed versus wild salmon. The first thing you should know is that farmed salmon is dyed pink. Yeah. Dyed. It is not naturally that beautiful pink color you see in your fishmonger's case. That color is achieved by an artificial dye, also known as a chemical, that tints the fish's flesh a color that is more appealing. I don't know about you, but that just makes my stomach turn. Turns out the natural color of farmed salmon is gray. Which is just gross. Farmed salmon eats a diet of prepared fish food and live their lives in big bodies of contained water. They don't swim around much, so they get really fat really fast, which helps the bottom lines.

Wild salmon is naturally a beautiful soft-pink color. It swims and breeds and just, in general, has the life that every fish would want. There are no chemicals used to dye their flesh and you don't need to worry about any sort of preservatives or anything else like that in your wild salmon. Yes, it may not be always available in your area, or you may have to get it canned or frozen, but it is so much better than eating farmed salmon. And yes, again, it can be a little more expensive. But since you are buying in bulk, cooking in batches, taking advantage of sales, and saving a dime where you can, spending a little extra on the quality stuff will not eliminate your savings.

So yeah, I included a little food ethics with your money-saving tips, but there was a method here: you got twice the information than you bargained for! And that's what happens when you shop smart and you shop ethically. Not only do you get to save some actual money, but you can then afford to go and get protein that is ethically sourced and tastes so much better than the factory farmed garbage most of us eat normally.

In the next chapter, I am going to give you thirty recipes for you to use all of that quality stuff you just bought. I am giving you ten breakfast recipes, ten dinner recipes, and ten dessert recipes. Yes, dessert! It's important to have some variety in your diet. Because when you get bored, you get frustrated. When you get frustrated, you get angry with your diet. And when you get angry with your diet, you end up binging, feeling guilty, and then going back to your diet like a dog who ran away from home and rolled in something smelly.

Don't be like that dog. Just eat some dessert every once in a while that follows the guidelines that I set out below and you will be able to have sustainable weight loss that you can maintain over your life.

Chapter 9: 30 Easy Carnivore/Keto Recipes

In this section, we are going to give you 30 recipes to follow on this diet. These recipes are on the ketogenic side of things, so if you want to go pure carnivore, make sure that you just eliminate any of the carbohydrates that are in the recipes. We are going to give you 10 full breakfast recipes, 10 dinner recipes, and 10 dessert (yes, dessert) recipes.

Breakfast:

1. Easy-peasy egg and cheese sandwiches:
These are great for a quick bite in the morning when you don't have time to be slaving over a hot stove.
Ingredients:

- Half a pound of ground breakfast sausage, out of the casings (I usually don't season this stuff, as it's already usually pretty high in sodium)
- Six eggs, scrambled
- Shredded cheddar jack cheese
- A few pats of butter
- Salt and pepper, to taste

Method:

- Form six patties with the breakfast sausage, about the size of your palm

- After you thoroughly wash your hands, preheat a medium sized skillet over medium high heat
- Melt the butter in the pan. When it foams up, cook the patties in the pan, about five minutes per side, until there is no more pink in the middle of the patties.
- Remove the patties from the pan and allow them to cool on a plate.
- Pour the scrambled eggs in the pan and cook for a few minutes, until the eggs are no longer liquid.
- Line up three of the sausage patties on a platter and top with the eggs and shredded cheese
- Top with the remaining patties
- Enjoy!

2. Healthy Toad in a Hole:

This is a great recipe when you want to add a little pizzazz to your morning eggs and maybe get your kids to eat a vegetable or two.

Ingredients:

- Yellow bell pepper
- Red bell pepper
- Green bell pepper
- Three eggs, whole
- Olive oil
- Salt and pepper, to taste

Method:

- With a sharp knife, cut off the top of the bell peppers
- Rip out the seeds
- Carefully run your knife along the inside of the bell peppers to remove the ribs
- Then cut the bell peppers into rounds (the eggs are going inside the pepper rings)
- Preheat a medium skillet over medium heat and put a drizzle of olive oil in there
- Sauté the pepper rings until they are beginning to soften, about four minutes
- Crack an egg in each pepper ring
- Cook the eggs until the white is opaque and the centers don't move
- Season with salt and pepper and serve

3. Jalapeno and egg bacon cups

Easy, spicy, and filling these are great to make a big batch of and then reheat to make a great breakfast on the run.

Ingredients:

- 6 slices of bacon
- Shredded mozzarella (to taste)
- Shredded Monterey jack cheese (to taste)
- 5 large eggs
- ¼ cup of sour cream
- 1 finely chopped jalapeno pepper

Method:

- Scramble the eggs together, adding salt and pepper as needed
- Mix in the jalapeno peppers, shredded cheese, and sour cream
- Line six muffin wells with the bacon
- Pour in the egg mixture
- Bake in a 375 degree oven for about 20 minutes

4. Healthy Breakfast Hash

What's not to love about a good hash in the morning. It's easy to prepare, it makes plenty for leftovers, and it's easy on the wallet to boot.

Ingredients:

- 1 bag (12 oz) of Brussels sprouts
- 6 slices of bacon, chopped roughly
- Four large eggs
- Olive oil
- Butter
- Salt and pepper to taste
- Shredded mozzarella cheese, for topping

Method:

- Thoroughly wash the Brussels sprouts to remove any sand and dirt from the leaves
- Remove the tough outer leaves of the sprouts
- Quarter the sprouts

- Heat up the olive oil and butter in a large skillet until sizzling
- Toss in the bacon and cook until crispy
- Pour off some of the rendered fat from the pan, reserve for later use in a future recipe
- Throw in the Brussels sprouts and sauté until they begin to take on some color and get a little caramelized around the edges
- Reintroduce the bacon into the pan
- Make some space in the pan for the eggs
- Crack the eggs in and cook until whites of the eggs are opaque
- Top with the shredded cheese and pop into a 400 degree oven for about three minutes, or until the cheese is bubbling on top.

5. Low Carb Breakfast Pizza

This recipe takes the idea of eating pizza for breakfast to a whole new level. It requires 10 minutes of preparation and 30 minutes to cook. It makes 8 servings and can be refrigerated for 5 days or frozen for 60 days.

Ingredients:

- ¼ tsp. pepper
- ½ C. heavy cream
- ½ tsp. salt
- 1 C. shredded cheese of choice

- 12 eggs
- 2 C. sliced peppers
- 8 ounces of sausage

Method:
- Ensure your oven is preheated to 350 degrees.
- Microwave peppers for 3 minutes.
- In a cast iron skillet, brown sausage. Set to the side.
- Mix pepper, salt, cream, and eggs together and place in skillet.
- Cook 5 minutes till the sides begin to become firm.
- Place skillet in over and back 15 minutes. Remove from oven.
- Add cheese, peppers, and sausage to skillet and place under broiler for 3 minutes.
- Allow to sit for 5 minutes to cool. Devour right away or split between meal prep containers.

6. The Dreamy Breakfast Tower

This is a creamy, dreamy, breakfast dish. It's super simple to make and packed with lots of protein and good fats to keep you satisfied for hours.

Ingredients:
- 4 large eggs
- 2 avocadoes, pitted and diced
- 1 red onion, diced
- 1 tomato, diced

- 1 jalapeno, seeded and diced
- Half a pound of ground sausage meat

Method:

- Form four patties of the sausage meat and set aside
- After thoroughly washing your hands, take a medium skillet and add a splash of olive oil
- Heat over medium heat until oil begins to shimmer
- Meanwhile, mash up the avocado and mix in the red onion, tomato, and jalapeno. Then add in a dash of olive oil, some salt, and some pepper
- Once the pan is heated, fry up your sausage
- Cook for approximately 5-6 minutes per side, until there is no more pink meat in the middle; remove the patties and set aside
- Then, cook your eggs sunny side up – this should take approximately five minutes
- Top your sausage patty with a few tablespoons of your avocado mixture and then put the egg on.
- Sprinkle with some salt and pepper and enjoy!

7. Bacon and Egg Roll-Ups

Is there anything better in the morning than bacon and eggs? Yes! Bacon, eggs, and cheese! Talk about a trifecta. These rollups are easy to prepare and take only a few minutes. Let's get started!

Ingredients:

- Four large eggs
- Half a cup of shredded sharp cheddar
- 12 strips of bacon
- Salt
- Pepper
- A few pats of butter
- A splash of milk or cream

Method:

- Preheat a skillet over medium heat with a few pats of butter
- While your pan is preheating, whisk your eggs with some salt, pepper, and a splash of milk or cream
- Once the pan is properly heated, pour the eggs in and cook for about 3 minutes, or until they are no longer liquid and hold their shape
- Lay out three slices of bacon on a sheet pan and make sure that they overlap
- Sprinkle the slices with some of the shredded cheese
- Top with some of the eggs and roll up
- Repeat with the rest of the bacon, eggs, and cheese
- Once you have all of your roll ups made, cook in that skillet until the bacon is crispy and the cheese is melted.
- Enjoy!

8. Eggs in Purgatory

We all have those mornings when maybe we have partied a little too hard the night before, or maybe we just need something a little more substantial before we head off to work. This recipe is full of protein, great fats, and some veggies. Like we said before, if you want to make it pure carnivore, just add some chicken and forego the veggies. But we think you'll like this recipe just as it is.

Ingredients:

- 1 8oz can of crushed tomatoes
- 1 jalapeno, diced
- Crushed red pepper flakes, about ½ teaspoon
- 2 scallions, diced small
- 2 tbsp. olive oil
- 4 large eggs

Method:

- Heat the olive oil in a medium skillet until it shimmers
- Add in the crushed tomatoes, crushed red pepper flakes, jalapeno, and cook until everything thickens, about 15 minutes
- Make four holes in the mixture and crack the eggs in there
- Cook the eggs until the whites are firm and the yolk is set, about five or so minutes
- Sprinkle with the chopped scallions and enjoy!

9. Eggs in Heaven

We figured that you might want some eggs that are just heavenly. These eggs are baked in a beautiful nest of egg whites, ham, and Parmesan cheese. They're perfectly fluffy and packed with protein and fat – and these are perfectly carnivorous. So enjoy!

Ingredients:

- Four eggs, whites, and yolks separated
- Chopped up ham
- ¼ cup of grated Parmesan cheese
- Finely chopped basil

Method:

- Preheat your oven to 450 degrees
- Whisk your eggs whites until they reach a stiff peak, about four minutes (use a hand mixer for this, unless you really want to work on those forearm muscles)
- Once you get your whites all whipped, fold in your Parmesan cheese, ham, and basil.
- Dollop the whites into four mounds on a greased cookie sheet
- Pop them into the oven for about three minutes
- Then, take the sheet out and carefully place the yolks into the mounds
- Bake for another three minutes and sprinkle with more Parmesan
- Enjoy!

10. Steak and eggs

This is a breakfast meant for royalty. I mean, a thick, juicy steak and a beautiful runny egg? What sounds better? Nothing, that's right.

Ingredients:

- Butter
- Bone-in ribeye steak
- One egg
- Salt
- Pepper

Method:

- Properly salt and pepper the steak
- Allow to rest at room temperature for at least 30 minutes, but no longer than an hour.
- Get your pan nice and hot
- Place your steak in the pan (preferably cast-iron)
- Do not move that steak for four and a half minutes
- Then, gently flip over and finish cooking for another four minutes.
- Once you flip that steak to finish cooking, put in your butter and gently baste your steak as it finishes cooking
- Once your steak is done, remove it and let it rest for at least ten minutes
- While your steak is resting, cook your egg sunny side up (about five minutes)
- Serve with the egg on top
- Enjoy!

Dinner

Now let's talk about dinner. Dinner is going to be one of your chances to really pull out the big guns and wow yourself and your family with some really great recipes. What follows is ten recipes for dinner that is full of good fats and protein, along with some veggies if you like. Read on!

1. Shrimp scampi with zucchini zoodles

We all know how "zoodles" have taken the food world by storm in the last few years. So this recipe uses zucchini noodles instead of pasta for this delicious shrimp scampi. It comes together in minutes and will fill you up for hours.

Ingredients:

- Half a pound of shrimp, peeled and deveined
- Three cloves of garlic, peeled
- 3 tbsp. olive oil
- 1 package zucchini zoodles
- 1 tbsp. red pepper flakes
- Juice of 1 lemon
- Salt
- Pepper

Method:

- Heat olive oil in a skillet
- When it's shimmering, add in your zucchini
- Cook for about 3 minutes, until the vegetables are soft, and season with salt, pepper, and red pepper flakes

- Use a zester and grate the garlic into the zoodles, cook for a further 60 seconds and be careful not to burn the carlic
- Then add in the shrimp and cook until they are a beautiful pink
- Pour in the lemon juice and stir everything together
- Serve and enjoy

2. Roasted chicken

Everyone should know how to properly roast a chicken. This is a skill that will serve you well in life because so few people know how to achieve that beautifully crispy skin on a chicken. The best part about a roasted chicken is that it takes only a few ingredients and some time in the oven to make a beautiful meal. Also, please remember to wash your hands each and every time you touch the chicken. Nobody wants salmonella. Ingredients:

- 1 four pound roasting chicken (do not get a fryer or any other kind of chicken – make sure it is a roasting hen)
- Salt
- Pepper
- Butter
- 2 lemons sliced thinly
- Olive oil

Method:

- Preheat your oven to 425 degrees

- Prepare a cookie sheet: line it with foil and place a rack on top – something that you would use to cool cookies on or a roasting rack, whichever you have.
- Now, time to get the chicken ready to go in the oven
- Make sure that all the giblets are taken out of the cavity and get ready to season like your life depends on it.
- Drizzle olive oil all over the chicken and give it a massage. Season generously with salt and pepper (INCLUDING THE CAVITY! People always forget this step – you really need to season the inside of your chicken.)
- Then, rub some butter under the skin and on top of the chicken
- Place some lemon slices in the cavity of the chicken
- Place some lemon slices on top of the chicken body
- Tie the legs together and tuck the wings under the body of the chicken (this will help the chicken cook evenly and quickly.)
- Place the chicken inside the oven and roast, breast side up, for at least an hour, or until the leg juices run clear.

3. Pan-roasted duck breast with butternut squash

This is a beautifully simple dish with flavors that just sing. It comes together very quickly and tastes absolutely amazing. It takes a little time, but it is so worth it in the end, I promise.

Ingredients:
- 2 duck breasts
- 1 butternut squash, diced

- Olive oil
- Salt
- Pepper

Method:
- Preheat your oven to 450 degrees
- Slather your diced butternut squash in olive oil and season generously with salt and pepper (and a little cinnamon, if you're feeling adventurous)
- Throw it on a sheet pan and roast for about half an hour to 40 minutes, or until the squash is fork-tender
- Meanwhile, cook your duck:
  - Deeply score the fat on the duck breasts with a paring knife
  - Season generously with salt and pepper
  - Place FAT SIDE DOWN in a COLD pan
    - If you place the duck in a hot pan, the fat will seal up and never render. Which means it will never cook and raw duck fat is just...not appetizing. So please, listen to me here and put your duck in a cold pan.
  - Gradually increase the heat until the fat begins to render from the duck breast
  - When the fat side is rendered and golden brown, flip the duck breast over to finish cooking – about another five minutes or so.
- Slice and serve with the butternut squash!

4. Grilled chicken hearts and livers

Remember how we talked about organ meats being great sources of micronutrients? Yeah, we really believe in that, so here is a recipe for organ meat kabobs that is easy and tasty.

Ingredients:

- Half a pound of chicken hearts
- Half a pound of chicken livers
- Salt
- Pepper
- Metal kabob skewers

Method:

- Generously salt and pepper the livers and hearts
- Thread onto the metal skewers
- Grill until done!
  - The livers and hearts should take about 2-3 minutes per side

5. Burger bombs

These are an easy way to get in some really great protein and a good amount of fat. Plus, they're really tasty, so there's that.

Ingredients:

- One pound of grass fed ground beef
- Garlic powder
- Salt

- Pepper
- Cubed sharp cheddar cheese

Method:

- Preheat your oven to 375 degrees
- Mix the ground beef with the garlic powder, salt, and pepper
- Form small patties the place and place a cube of cheese in the middle
- Close the meat to surround the cheese block
- Bake in the oven on a cookie sheet for about 15 minutes.
- Serve!

6. Flat iron steak with caramelized onions

This is another easy recipe filled with good fats and lots of protein. The caramelized onions provide a nice hint of sweetness with the salty and meaty flavors of the steak.

Ingredients:

- 1 flatiron steak, fresh from the butcher
- Olive oil
- Salt
- Pepper
- Juice of 1 lime
- Chopped cilantro, for garnish
- 3 Vidalia onions, sliced

Method:

- Thinly slice the onions while the olive oil heats up in a skillet
- Add the onions to the pan and cook slowly over medium, or medium-low heat until the onions are beautifully brown and sweet
- While the onions are caramelizing, season your steak and leave out at room temperature
- Scrape the onions out of the pan and leave the "fond", or the beautiful little brown bits, in the pan. This will help add flavor to the steak.
- Pour a little more olive oil in your pan and let it heat up
- Add the steak to the pan and cook for about three minutes, then flip and cook for another 2-3 minutes
- Slice, top with the onions, and enjoy!

7. Oven-roasted Salmon with Pesto

This is a great recipe for a week night dinner when you just don't have a lot of time to slave over a hot stove. It comes together in about 45 minutes from start to finish, and will make lots for leftovers! Pair it with one of your favorite veggies or just enjoy on its own if you are looking to keep it more carnivore-friendly.

Ingredients:

- 1 pound skin-on salmon fillets, cut into 6 ounce portions
- 3 cups basil leaves
- ½ cup pine nuts, unsalted

- Olive oil
- Salt
- Pepper
- Grated pecorino Romano cheese, about ½ a cup, more to taste

Method:

- Blend basil, pine nuts, and cheese in a blender while you drizzle in olive oil
- Keep an eye on it and add oil until it forms a loose paste
- Salt and pepper it to taste
- Preheat your oven to 450 degrees
- Place the salmon fillets on a baking sheet lined with parchment paper, skin side down
- Slather the tops of the fillets with the pesto
- Sprinkle with more cheese
- Roast in the oven for approximately 12-15 minutes
- Enjoy!

8. Pan-roasted scallops with asparagus

This is another great recipe for a meal that comes together in minutes. It is quick, healthy, and packed with lots of protein, high-quality fats, and fiber-filled veggies. Get ready to have a restaurant worthy dish in a matter of minutes.

Ingredients:

- Small scallops, about a pound's worth
- Salt

- Pepper
- Olive oil
- Asparagus, woody ends trimmed off

Method:
- Preheat your oven to 375 degrees
- Toss your asparagus with olive oil, salt, and pepper
- Spread on a foil-lined baking sheet and pop in the oven for about 15 minutes
- Meanwhile, heat up about a tablespoon of olive oil in a pan over medium-high heat
- Right before you cook your scallops, season them generously with salt and pepper
- Sear on each side for 90 seconds
- Serve with the roasted asparagus and enjoy!

9. Roasted chicken thighs with tomato and jalapeno salsa

This is a tasty recipe that has bright and vivacious flavors sure to wake up your palate. It is high in fat and protein, with some tasty veggies in a supporting role. This is a quick recipe and does not involve a lot of prep or standing over the stove. The most involved part is chopping up everything for the salsa, but I promise the effort is worth it.

Ingredients:
- 1 pound chicken thighs, skin on
- Olive oil

- Salt
- Pepper
- Vinegar, to taste (this is for the salsa)
- 3 Roma tomatoes, diced
- 1 jalapeno, diced fine
- 3 cloves of garlic, grated
- Half of a red onion, diced
- Coconut oil

Method:

- Mix the tomatoes, jalapeno, garlic, onion, and enough olive oil and vinegar to make things moist and a little like a sauce
- Salt and pepper the salsa to your taste
- Set aside to allow the vinegar to marry with the other ingredients
- Preheat your oven to 375 degrees
- Next, mix up about a cup of coconut oil with a heavy heap of salt
- Shove that stuff under the skin of the chicken thighs
- Generously salt the skin of the thighs and drizzle with olive oil
- Roast the chicken in the oven for about 35-40 minutes, or until cooked through.
- Top the chicken with the salsa and dig in!

10. Perfect filet mignon with roasted mushroom sauce

I think this is probably the recipe you all were waiting for. When you are done with this recipe, you will have a perfectly cooked, medium-rare, filet mignon that is bathed in a buttery mushroom sauce. My mouth is watering just writing this recipe! Read on!

Ingredients:

- 2 filet mignons, about six ounces each
- Butter
- Salt
- Pepper
- Shitake mushrooms
- Garlic
- Thyme
- Sherry (not cooking sherry – go out and get the good stuff)

Method:

- About half an hour before you are ready to start cooking, set out your filet mignons on a counter (or somewhere where cats, children, or other hungry beings won't be tempted to mess with them) and generously salt and pepper them all over
- Preheat your oven to 325 degrees
- Toss shitake mushroom with olive oil, salt, and pepper and spread on a baking sheet lined with parchment paper. Top with a few sprigs of thyme and grate over a few cloves of garlic

- Roast in the oven for about 30 minutes, turning the mushrooms over after 20 minutes
- Remove from the oven and let rest while you cook your steaks.
- Preheat a cast iron pan over medium to medium-high heat
- Sear the filets for three minutes on each side (not just top and bottom, remember)
- Remove and add butter to the pan
- Toss in your mushrooms and a splash of brandy
- Reduce to a nice sauce
- Pour your mushrooms over your filets and enjoy!

Dessert

This is my favorite part of the meal. Like I said before, having dessert on this diet is not strictly carnivore. But I would rather have you enjoy this diet and way of eating and be able to make it a sustainable lifestyle for you.

1. Blueberry Tarts

Fruit tarts are my favorite desserts of all time. I love chocolate, don't get me wrong, but there is something about fruit that is mixed with salt, a little sugar, and butter that just gets my mouth watering every time. This recipe is keto friendly and absolutely delicious!

Ingredients:

For the crust, you will need:

- 1 ounce of butter, cold and cubed
- 1 tablespoon of cookie pieces (whatever kind you prefer, but I like pecan cookies for this recipe)
- ¼ of a cup almond flour
- 1 tablespoon of keto-friendly confectioner's sugar

For the filling, you will need:
- 1 ounce of butter, cubed
- 1 teaspoon lemon juice
- ½ tablespoon almond flour
- Fresh blueberries, about 40 grams
- 2 tablespoons keto-friendly sweetener

Method:
- Preheat the oven to 350 degrees
- Using a food processor, pulse the ingredients for the crust together until it forms a dough
- Press the dough into a tart pan that is four inches in diameter (yes, this makes individual tarts)
- Pierce the dough with a fork to prevent it from rising in the oven
- Blind bake your crust for 12 minutes
- Allow it to cool before adding the filling
- Mix together your blueberries, 1 and ½ tablespoons of sweetener as well as the almond flour and lemon juice
- Pour into cooled tart shell.
- Top with remaining butter and sweetener
- Bake at 350 degrees for 10 minutes

- Cool and eat!

2. Individual Pumpkin Tarts

Pumpkin is one of my favorite flavors of fall. Since the holidays always seem to be right around the corner, this is a great dessert to have on hand so that you don't overindulge in other sweet treats that are sure to be lurking around. Keep these on hand and you will have a healthy alternative no matter what comes your way!

Ingredients:

For the crust, you will need:

- 1 ounce of butter, cold and cubed
- 1 tablespoon of cookie pieces (whatever kind you prefer, but I like pecan cookies for this recipe)
- ¼ of a cup almond flour
- 1 tablespoon of keto-friendly confectioner's sugar

For the filling, you will need:

- A dash of ground ginger (get the fresh stuff, not the sawdust that is in your pantry right now.)
- Four tablespoons of pumpkin puree (pure pumpkin puree, not pumpkin pie filling from a manufacturer whom I cannot name due to legal reasons)
- 1 teaspoon pumpkin pie spice
- 3 tablespoons heavy whipping cream
- 2 tablespoons of keto-friendly brown sugar substitute

Method:
- Preheat the oven to 350 degrees
- Using a food processor, pulse the ingredients for the crust together until it forms a dough
- Press the dough into a tart pan that is four inches in diameter (yes, this makes individual tarts)
- Pierce the dough with a fork to prevent it from rising in the oven
- Blind bake your crust for 12 minutes
- Allow it to cool before adding the filling
- Blend all filling ingredients in a food processor
- Scrape filling into tart crust
- Bake for 12-15 minutes
- Chill for at least one hour before enjoying.

3. Chunky chocolate chip cookies

I love relaxing with a big chocolate chip cookie, a hot cup of coffee, and a good book. This is a great way to have that cookie without a heaping helping of guilt. These cookies are keto friendly and they taste absolutely amazing. Be prepared for minimal effort and maximum taste.

Ingredients:
- 1 teaspoon vanilla extract
- ¾ teaspoon baking powder
- ¼ cup chopped pecans
- 1/3 cup chocolate chips that are keto-friendly

- 1 egg
- 4 tablespoons of melted butter
- ¼ cup keto sugar substitute
- ¼ cup of pecan cookie pieces
- ½ cup of almond flour

Method:

- Preheat your oven to 350 and line a cookie sheet with non-stick aluminum foil
- Cream butter and sugar together as you add in the egg.
- Mix in the chocolate chips to your butter, sugar, and egg mixture
- Sift all dry ingredients together in a separate bowl
- Mix the dry ingredients into the wet and stir until just combined – do not over mix.
- Divide the dough into six even balls and place on cookie sheet
- Bake for approximately 15 minutes
- Allow to cool on a rack before devouring

4. Individual chocolate tarts

Who out there loves chocolate – raise your hand! I feel like it is one of those universally appealing ingredients. And honestly, if you don't like chocolate, I don't know if we can be friends. Sorry, but I feel very strongly about this issue. I almost left my son's father when he told me he refused to eat ketchup, so I clearly have emotional ties to food preferences. Luckily, he also loves chocolate and doesn't gag when I put ketchup on stuff, so we are still going strong, but it was a scary time there for a while. Anyway, what follows here is a recipe for individual chocolate tarts that you can make for yourself and your partner in crime.

Ingredients:

For the crust, you will need:

- 1 ounce of butter, cold and cubed
- 1 tablespoon of cookie pieces (whatever kind you prefer, but I like pecan cookies for this recipe)
- ¼ of a cup almond flour
- 1 tablespoon of keto-friendly confectioner's sugar

For the filling, you will need:

- 28 grams of keto-friendly chocolate chips
- 1 tablespoon butter
- ½ teaspoon vanilla extract
- ½ tablespoon keto-friendly confectioner's sugar
- 2 tablespoons heavy whipping cream

Method:

- Preheat the oven to 350 degrees
- Using a food processor, pulse the ingredients for the crust together until it forms a dough
- Press the dough into a tart pan that is four inches in diameter (yes, this makes individual tarts)
- Pierce the dough with a fork to prevent it from rising in the oven

- Blind bake your crust for 12 minutes
- Allow it to cool before adding the filling
- For the filling, simply heat all ingredients over low heat in a saucepan until it comes together
- Pour into the cooled tart shell and chill until filling is set
- Devour!

5. Pecan Cookies

I hope you're starting to notice a theme here. These recipes are meant to be quick and easy – a way for you to make yourself dessert when you just need something sweet and don't want to wait any longer than you have to. Plus, cookies and tarts are familiar – I'm not going to have you make chia pudding or some weird version of a keto dessert that you don't recognize. Hopefully, this will make your transition into the carnivore lifestyle a little easier.

Ingredients:

- ¼ teaspoon of salt
- ¼ teaspoon of vanilla
- ¼ cup keto-friendly sugar substitute
- 1/5 cup chopped, toasted pecans
- 5 tablespoons butter, melted
- 1/3 cup pecan cookie bits
- 2/3 cup of almond flour

Method:

- Combine all ingredients in a large bowl and mix until everything comes together
- Preheat your oven to 350 degrees
- Separate dough into six even balls
- Place on a cookie sheet lined with aluminum foil
- Bake for approximate 12 minutes
- Place on a rack to cool
- Eat!

6. Chocolate Mug Cake

Who doesn't like an individual cake that you can just make in a mug? And especially one that comes together in just minutes? This is a great recipe for when you just need something sweet and don't want to take more than a few minutes. It's also great for when you just don't feel like sharing dessert. I know what that's like – my son always has to have exactly what I'm having. So when he goes to bed, this is my favorite thing to make for myself. I can sit down with a cup of tea and just enjoy a little bit of sweetness with my peace and quiet.

Ingredients:

- 15 grams chopped pecans or nuts of your choice
- ½ teaspoon of baking powder
- 2 tablespoons of keto-friendly chocolate chips
- ½ teaspoon of vanilla
- 2 tablespoons of pecan cookie bits

103

- 1 egg
- 2 tablespoons keto-friendly sugar substitute
- 3 tablespoons of butter
- 2 tablespoons of cocoa powder
- 3 tablespoons of almond flour

Method:
- In a microwave-safe mug, melt the butter
- Mix your sugar substitute into the melted butter
- After that, add in the rest of your ingredients and mix well
- Microwave for two minutes
- Let cool for about sixty seconds and then enjoy!

7. Peanut Butter Pie

I'm pretty sure my partner loves the combination of peanut butter and chocolate almost more than he loves me. In fact, we might be tied, except for the fact that I helped produce a pretty cute kid. So I think I'm safe for now. But man, this peanut butter and chocolate pie is pretty darn amazing, if I do say so myself. I hope that you enjoy it and maybe share it with your partner, though I totally understand if you keep it all to yourself. I won't tell anyone.

Ingredients:

For the crust, you will need:
- ¼ cup cocoa powder
- 5 tablespoons keto sugar substitute

- 4 ounces of melted butter
- ¾ cup of almond flour
- 1 cup of pecan cookie bits

For the filling, you will need:
- ¾ cup creamy peanut butter, preferably organic
- ½ cup keto-friendly sugar substitute
- 4 ounces of softened cream cheese
- 1/3 cup of whipped cream

Method:
- Pulse all the ingredients for the crust in a food processor
- Dump out into a 9" pie pan and use your fingers to even everything out and press the crust into the corners and up the sides
- Use an electric mixer to whip the heavy cream into soft peaks before mixing in the rest of the ingredients.
- Pour the filling into the crust and chill for at least four hours.
- Then slice and enjoy!

8. Chocolate-chip Cheesecake

My partner also loves cheesecake. Man, he will just go to town on one of these bad boys. He always demands cheesecake instead of regular cake for his birthdays, and I earn major brownie points when I make him a chocolate chip version of a cheesecake. He just can't stop himself. It's actually pretty cute. Anyway, he also follows this carnivore lifestyle with me, so when he wants to indulge but also doesn't want to wreck his progress and feel sick, I make him one of these.

Ingredients:

For the crust, you will need:

- 1 cup of those familiar pecan cookie bits
- 4 ounces of melted butter
- 1 cup of almond flour
- 5 tablespoons of keto-friendly sugar substitute
- 2/3 cup of keto-friendly chocolate chips

For the filling, you will need:

- 1 and ½ teaspoons of vanilla
- ¾ cup of keto-friendly chocolate chips
- 1/3 cup heavy whipping cream
- 3 eggs
- 24 ounces of cream cheese (FULL FAT)
- 1 cup keto-friendly sugar substitute

Method:

- Pulse the cookie bits, almond flour, and sugar substitute in a food processor
- Add in the butter and pulse again until a dough forms
- Once that dough forms, turn it out into a bowl and stir in the keto-friendly chocolate chips.
- Press dough into a 9" springform pan.
- Pierce the bottom of the crust several times with a fork and bake in a 350 degree oven for approximately 12 minutes

- Remove from the oven and allow to cool while you prepare the filling
- To make the filling, cream together all ingredients, save the chocolate chips, using an electric mixer.
- Once it all comes together, add in ½ cup of the chips and mix
- Pour into the prebaked shell and then sprinkle the remaining chocolate chips over the top
- Bake the cheesecake at 315 degrees for about 1 hour and 15 minutes
- Remove from oven and allow to cool.
- Refrigerate for 24 hours before enjoying.

9. Pound cake with lemon frosting

This is definitely not your mama's pound cake. Instead of a cake that is filled with an unhealthy amount of flour and sugar, this is a healthy take that still tastes delicious and satisfies that itch for pound cake. I personally enjoy this cake toasted for breakfast with a little bit of butter. It's absolutely delicious and will fill you up for hours because of its healthy fats. Read on for a simple recipe that is sure to please!

Ingredients:

For the cake, you will need:

- ½ teaspoon salt
- 1 teaspoon baking powder
- 1 and ½ teaspoons vanilla extract
- 2 tablespoons of lemon juice

- 8 ounces of cream cheese
- 1 cup of keto-friendly sugar substitute
- 6 room temperature eggs
- ½ cup of softened butter
- 2 cups of almond flour

For the icing, you will need:
- 1 tablespoon of lemon juice
- 1/3 cup of keto-friendly confectioner's sugar
- Four ounces of cream cheese

Method:
- For the cake, start by preheating the oven to 350 degrees
- Mix the lemon juice and sugar substitute in a large bowl until it resembles mush
- Add in the eggs, softened cream cheese, softened butter, and vanilla. Cream until smooth.
- Sift the dry ingredients into another bowl
- Slowly add in the dry ingredients to the wet
- Pour the mixture into a greased bread loaf pan
- Bake the cake for approximately 50 minutes, or until a toothpick inserted into the middle comes up clean
- While the cake cools, make the icing:
  - Cream together all frosting ingredients with an electric mixer
  - Once the cake is removed from loaf pan and is completely cool, pour icing over

o   Allow icing to set and then enjoy!

10. Key Lime Pie

Okay, so our final recipe is going to be key lime pie. I decided to include this recipe because key lime pie is my ultimate dessert, whether it is winter, summer, fall, spring, whatever. I love key lime pie. I love the sharp sour notes of the key limes that contrast with the fat from the butter and sweetness from the sugar substitutes. It is such a perfect flavor combination. So I wanted to end the recipe section of the book with my absolute favorite recipe. So here we go!

Ingredients:

For the crust, you will need:

- 2 tablespoons of keto-friendly sugar substitute
- 1/3 cup of butter, melted
- ½ cup of almond flour
- ¾ cup of pecan cookie bits

For the filling, you will need:

- 1 teaspoon xanthan gum (a thickener)
- 1 cup of sour cream (full fat!)
- 1 cup keto-friendly confectioner's sugar
- ¾ cup of dried milk powder
- 1 cup of juice from key limes (it is important that they are key limes, not regular limes)
- 1 cup of heavy whipping cream

Method:

- Pulse all the ingredients for the crust in a food processor
- Press the crust into a 9 inch spring form pan
- Bake in a 350 degree oven for approximately 8 minutes
- Allow to cool while you prepare the filling
- Blend together all filling ingredients
- Pour into cooled crust and bake in the oven for about 13 minutes
- Allow to cool on a rack for at least one hour
- Place in refrigerator and allow to set for 24 hours
- Then, slice and enjoy!

Okay, so that wraps up our recipes section of the book. I hope you find these recipes useful and tasty. Good luck!

Final Thoughts

We have spent a lot of time together, and I have to say, I have truly enjoyed writing this book. It really has been quite a labor of love. I enjoy talking about food and health, so when I get a chance to write about both, it truly makes me excited. I hope that you were inspired by this excitement and are ready to embark on a journey to change your life.

Change is never easy. I speak from personal experience with this. When I was twenty two years old, I was the heaviest I have ever been in my life. I was a junior in college, majoring in finance, and just generally unhappy with my life. I knew that I was unhealthy – not only was I overweight (which we will talk about in a minute), but I was always tired, I got sick very easily, and I could never seem to concentrate on things for a long period of time.

So one day I just decided that I was going to step on the scale and face the truth. I looked down at that number and I just burst into tears. I weighed 240 pounds. I was a 5 foot, two inch female who weighed 240 pounds. This is nearly twice of what I should weigh! After I dried my tears, I called my doctor and made a plan. I was going to lose this weight and I was going to get healthy. Nothing was going to get in my way.

I went shopping for food, I cleared out my dorm room of any kind of crappy food and started cooking my own meals. I focused on protein, healthy fats, and veggies. I controlled my carbohydrate consumption to the gram. I also visited the gym on a daily basis. I never once missed a workout or had a cheat meal. I ended up losing seventy pounds purely by diet and exercise. It was amazing.

I was able to prove to myself that my mind and determination was stronger than any outside force. Unfortunately, life hit back hard. I decided to go to graduate school. I met my partner, I ended up having a child. And while these are all great things to happen, it also had a very negative effect on my waistline. The stress from school caused me to forget about my eating habits. And since I was in a relationship that of course meant a lot of eating out and celebratory meals.

Pregnancy didn't help either! I ended up gaining back about 30 of those pounds. I was so depressed. I had such success and then I just ended up failing. I was so down on myself and found myself in this awful downward spiral. But then I found the carnivore diet. It was something I could do without a lot of effort and planning, which was a big plus to me, since I have a toddler. Planning and effort goes out the window for moms when they have a toddler.

It was also a diet that didn't require me to count calories or weigh my food. As someone who has a borderline obsessive relationship with food that is sometimes very unhealthy, it sounded like a good way to lose weight without losing my mind. Plus, my boyfriend loves steak and my two year old doesn't really much care what's on his plate as long as Elmo is on the television, so I had my work cut out for me.

I shopped for the food, I made the food, at the food, and went back to the gym. It took a few weeks to get used to this new way of eating and I fell a few times during the beginning of the process, but I am happy to say that I lost those thirty pounds I gained back. And now I am working on losing the rest. I plan on getting to a healthy weight with this diet.

I haven't seen any ill effects on my health; all of my bloodwork comes back stellar. I am less tired, my head is clearer, and clothes are fitting better. I am looking forward to continuing on this diet and losing more weight until I am finally at a healthy body weight. See, this diet has helped me see that I love myself as I am. I think I'm beautiful. My boyfriend thinks I'm beautiful. And my son thinks that the sun rises and sets with me. My impetus on this journey is not to love myself more but is rather to simply get to a healthy weight and maintain it.

I want to grow old with my boyfriend. I want to see my son get married. I want to experience grandchildren one day. And while there are a lot of other factors dealing with my longevity that I cannot control, one thing I can control is what I put into my body and how often I exercise. So by taking control of my diet and exercise, I can make sure that I will be around for a really long time.

I wanted to share this story with you because I want you to understand that the person writing this book is human. I understand the struggle and that's why I wrote this book – I want to help you struggle less. I hope that this book gives you enough tips and tricks and recipes to get you through the rough parts of your journey and sets you up for smooth sailing. So I wish you all the best!

CPSIA information can be obtained
at www.ICGtesting.com
Printed in the USA
LVHW080121171020
668893LV00004B/563